# CYTOLOGY AND SURGICAL PATHOLOGY OF GYNECOLOGIC NEOPLASMS

# CURRENT CLINICAL PATHOLOGY

ANTONIO GIORDANO, MD, PHD

*SERIES EDITOR*

For further titles published in this series, go to
http://www.springer.com/springer/series/7632

# Cytology and Surgical Pathology of Gynecologic Neoplasms

Edited by

## David Chhieng, MD, MBA, MSHI

*Yale University School of Medicine, New Haven, CT, USA*

## Pei Hui, MD, PhD

*Yale University School of Medicine, New Haven, CT, USA*

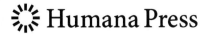 Humana Press

*Editors*
David Chhieng
Department of Pathology
Yale University School of Medicine
New Haven, CT
USA
david.chhieng@yale.edu

Pei Hui
Department of Pathology
Yale University School of Medicine
New Haven, CT
USA
pei.hui@yale.edu

ISBN 978-1-60761-163-9        e-ISBN 978-1-60761-164-6
DOI 10.1007/978-1-60761-164-6
Springer New York Dordrecht Heidelberg London

Library of Congress Control Number: 2010937989

Springer is part of Springer Science+Business Media (www.springer.com)

# Preface

The neoplasms found in the female genital tract are numerous and diagnostically growing more complex. Understanding gynecological pathology can be overwhelming. As an extension to comprehensive textbooks that are ubiquitous around sign-out microscope, this text has been written to provide a practical reference for practicing pathologists and cytopathologists in a quick and concise fashion. The primary focus of our book is on gynecological tumors, specifically common ones and their benign mimics, and every effort is made to integrate major diagnostic criteria with the ancillary studies. We hope we have made concrete the usually abstract dictum of gynecological pathology on both histological and cytological grounds. Understandably, as one of the highly complex pathology specialties, it is impossible to include every aspect of its ingredients in this compact reference book. Hematoxylin and eosin staining and immunohistochemistry remain the cornerstones of diagnostic gynecological pathology. This manual presents a logical approach to pathological diagnosis based primarily on conventional histology and cytology and assembles the most important diagnostic features of common neoplastic entities of the female genital tract. The most common differential diagnosis is discussed when necessary. Many entities in gynecological pathology may have multiple names and variants, but an attempt has been made to present a concise approach to the diagnostic problem often reflecting opinions of the authors.

Throughout the book, the approach is simple and straightforward entity-based discussion of each diagnostic entity followed by cytopathology related to the whole group of disease under each chapter. Because of this practical approach and the concrete and accessible nature of the material, we believe that this text also forms the basis for a bridge course to introduce residents, fellows, and junior practitioners to the specialty practice of gynecological pathology.

We wish to express our deepest gratitude to all of our mentors, past and current, who have been the major source of knowledge and courage in our academic careers. Our sincere appreciation goes to many colleagues and trainees in pathology at Yale University and University at Alabama, who have shared or presented many cases that provided the basis for this volume.

# Contents

# Chapter 1
# Normal Histology of Female Genital Organs

**Keywords** Normal • Histology • Cytology • Female genital tracts • The Bethesda system

## 1.1 Normal Histology of Vulva

The anatomy of vulva covers mons pubis, prepuce, frenulum, clitoris, labia minora, labia major, vulvar vestibule, urethral meatus, Bartholin's and Skene's glands, hymen, and introitus. Squamous epithelium covers surfaces of all vulvar structures. Mons pubis and labia major are covered by keratinizing squamous epithelium (skin) associated with all types of cutaneous adnexa, including hair follicles, sebaceous glands, apocrine glands, and sweat glands. Labia minor and inward to vaginal introitus and hymen are mainly covered by nonkeratinizing squamous epithelium associated with no or rare sweat and sebaceous glands. Bilateral Bartholin's glands are located posterolaterally in the vulvar vestibule and have tubuloalveolar structures, including acini of mucin-secreting columnar cells and ducts lined by transitional to squamous epithelium. There are also minor vestibular glands that are tubular and lined by mucin-secreting columnar cells. Skene's glands are also paired glandular structures covered by pseudostratified mucin-secreting columnar epithelium, located closely and posterolateral to the urethra. The clitoris is covered by nonkeratinizing squamous epithelium and contains stroma that is rich in erectile vascular structures similar to corpora cavernosa of the penis.

## 1.2 Normal Histology of Vagina

The vagina is a tubular organ consisting of stratified nonkeratinizing squamous mucosa, muscularis, and adventitia. The lamina propria is rich in elastic fiber and lymphovascular networks. The Gartner's duct (mesonephric remnant) is found along the lateral vaginal walls and is composed of clusters of small tubular glands surrounding a central duct. Luminal eosinophilic secretion is characteristic.

## 1.3 Normal Histology of Cervix

The cervix is anatomically divided into portio vaginalis that protrudes into the upper vagina and supravaginal portion. The portio vaginalis is further separated into ectocervix (outer surface) and endocervix (inner mucosal surface connecting the endocervical canal). The ectocervix is covered by nonkeratinizing stratified squamous epithelium and the endocervix is lined by mucinous epithelium in connection with underlying branching mucinous glands. The squamocolumnar junction between ectocervix and endocervix is the famous "transformation zone" (TZ), where the two types of epithelium move up and down replacing one another (metaplasia) depending on the age, hormonal, and reproductive status of a woman (Fig. 1.1). It is well known that the TZ is the most vulnerable anatomic site of the cervix to the development of various HPV-related malignant

D. Chhieng and P. Hui (eds.), *Cytology and Surgical Pathology of Gynecologic Neoplasms*,
Current Clinical Pathology, DOI 10.1007/978-1-60761-164-6_1,
© Springer Science+Business Media, LLC 2011

**Fig. 1.1** The transformation
zone of the cervix (H.E. ×40)

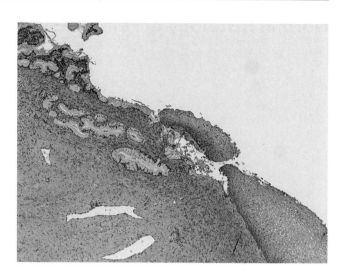

and premalignant conditions. When endocervical glandular epithelium moves onto the ectocervix, a grossly identifiable change as red erosion-like area occurs; this condition is referred to by the term "ectropion." Mucinous endocervical glandular epithelium covers the endocervical canal and merges with endometrial epithelium at the point where the uterine isthmus begins.

## 1.4 Normal Histology of Uterus

The uterus is a hollow organ divided into cervix and corpus. Above the inner openings of bilateral fallopian tubes, the superior portion of the corpus is the fundus. The portion where the distal corpus merges with the upper endocervical canal is the isthmus or lower uterine segment. The uterine cavity is triangular with an average length of 6 cm. The lining of the corpus is the endometrium. The thick myometrium constitutes the bulk of uterine mass. The outer surface of the uterus is covered by peritoneal serosa. The endometrium is histologically and functionally divided into superficial functionalis and deep basalis (Fig. 1.2). The hormonally regulated functionalis is further separated into the outer most compactum and the inner spongiosum. The basalis contains hormonally inactive reserve or stem cells. The stroma consists of endometrial stromal cells and rich vasculatures, both of which are hormonally responsive.

During the reproductive years, the endometrium undergoes cyclic morphologic and functional changes according to the ovulatory cycle. The cyclic alterations of the endometrium are divided into proliferative, secretory, and menstrual phases. In concert with the estrogen production during the ovarian follicular phase, the endometrial glands are proliferative and gradually increase in both number and size (from small straight tubular glands to large coiled glands in the late proliferative phase). The glands are covered by monolayer or pseudostratified, columnar epithelial cells with pencil-shaped nuclei. The cells are mitotically active. Scattered ciliated cells are present. The cellular stroma contains endometrial stromal cells that are small, round to oval with scant cytoplasm and round nuclei (Fig. 1.3). The thin-walled straight tubular vessels are characteristic for proliferative endometrium. During the secretory/progestin phase, the endometrial glands undergo daily predictable morphologic changes. The glands become serpentine to cystic to papillary cystic with cytoplasmic secretion (Fig. 1.4), typically subnuclear at day 17 and supranuclear at day 19 of a 28-day menstrual cycle. The endometrial stroma becomes edematous, reaching maximum at day 22. Stromal decidualization begins on day 23 and reaches its completion on day 26. Characteristic spiral arteriols cuffed by decidualized stromal cells begin to appear at day 23. When fertilization does not occur, the endometrium undergoes rapid degeneration, leading to menstrual

**Fig. 1.2** Low-power view of early proliferative endometrium, which is roughly divided into the superficial functionalis and deep basalis. Note somewhat irregular glands present in the basalis (H.E. ×20)

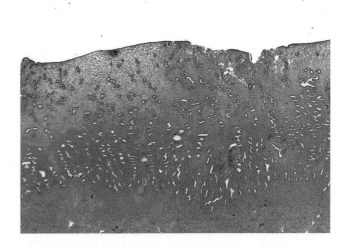

**Fig. 1.3** Proliferative endometrium. Note the early proliferative endometrial glands and the presence of evenly distributed spiral arteriols in the stroma (H.E. ×40)

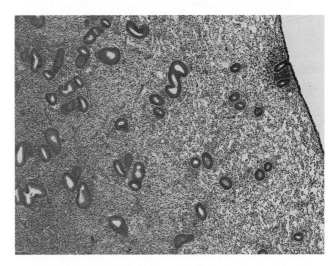

**Fig. 1.4** Late secretory phase endometrium (H.E. ×40)

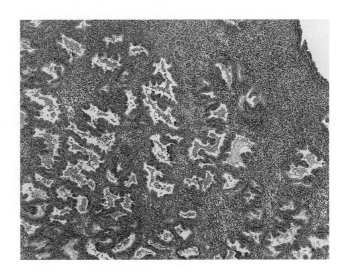

breakdown, which usually lasts 4–5 days. Menstrual endometrium is characterized by ruptured glands with secretory exhaustion, stromal condensation and collapse (stromal balls), vascular fibrin thrombi, and acute and chronic inflammatory cells. If fertilization occurs, the secretory endometrium will further evolve to prepare for implantation of the embryo into gestational hyperplastic endometrium, which is characterized by reappearance of both secretory endometrial glands and stromal edema, combined with enhanced predecidulization. Glands in the spongiosum may show the so-called Arias-Stella reaction by the presence of large atypical glandular cells with clear or eosinophilic cytoplasm and hyperchromatic and enlarged nuclei, some of which are epically positioned, simulating the hobnailed cells seen in a clear cell carcinoma. Similar cytologic changes can be seen in the epithelial cells in the cervix, fallopian tube, or endometriosis.

## 1.5  Normal Histology of Fallopian Tube

Fallopian tubes are paired tubular structures originating from the superolateral walls of the uterus, and run within the upper edges of broad ligaments. Anatomically, fallopian tubes are divided, from proximal to distal, into intramural (within the uterine wall), isthmus, ampulla, and infundibulum.

The distal abdominal ostium of infundibulum is configured by irregular figure-like structures, called fimbriae. The mucosa consists of overall longitudinal, yet branching folds or plicae that are covered by three types of epithelial cells: ciliated, secretory, and intercalating cells (Fig. 1.5). The muscularis propria consists of complete inner circular and outer longitudinal layers of smooth muscle. Walthard nests are common epithelial structures of urothelial differentiation within the wall of fallopian tube, mesosalpinx, mesovarium, or even ovarian hilar stroma.

## 1.6  Normal Histology of Ovary

Ovaries are paired oval organs that are 4.0 cm in average size. They are located inferoposterior to the fallopian tubes and connected to the broad ligament and uterine cornu by mesovarium and uteror-ovarian ligament, respectively. The surface of ovary is covered by a single layer of modified mesothelium of celomic nature, which is embryologically related to the lining of the entire mullerian ducts. Focal invagination of the surface epithelium creates cortical epithelial inclusions of less than 1.0 cm. The ovarian stroma is divided into cortex and medulla. Both compartments are composed of plump spindle cells of fibroblastic or myofibroblastic types, arranged in dense storiform patterns. There is a rich reticulum meshwork,

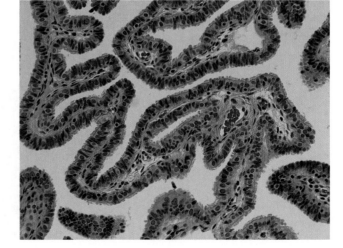

**Fig. 1.5** Fallopian tube mucosa at high power. The mucosa consists of overall longitudinal yet branching folds or plicae that are covered by three types of epithelial cells: ciliated, secretory, and intercalating cells (H.E. ×200)

particularly in the cortex, among stromal cells. Luteinized stromal cells with bubbly clear cytoplasm may be seen in singles or clusters. Bundles of smooth muscle fibers, nests of adipose cells, or even endometrial stromal cells may be present as well. Ovarian germ cells or follicles at various maturation stages are present in the cortex of ovary in women before menopause (Fig. 1.6). Primordial follicles consist of one germ cell surrounded by a flattened single layer of granulosa cells. Maturing follicles are typically composed of an oocyte surrounded by a varying number of granulosa cells and an outer layer of theca cells. Call-Exner bodies are round cavitary arrangement of granulosa cells with central accumulation of eosinophilic PAS-positive filamentous basal lamina. Mitoses, sometimes numerous, may be found in the granulosa and theca cells of a secondary follicle. The outer theca layer is further separated to luteinized, well-delineated theca interna and an outer less distinct theca externa. The central ovarian medulla consists of cellular stroma and developing follicles before adolescence, or corpora albican embedded in a meshwork of blood vessels in an adult woman. The hilum of the ovary is rich in blood vessels of various calibers. Clusters of hilum cells resembling Leydig cells in testis are frequently found in the hilar region, so is rete ovarii (irregular, interconnecting clefts, tubules, or cysts lined by flat to cuboidal epithelial cells and surrounded by a cuff of spindle cell ovarian-type stromal cells).

## 1.7 Normal Cytology of Female Genital Tract Organs

### 1.7.1 Squamous Cells

The predominant cell type in a Pap test is squamous cell. There are three types of squamous cells: superficial, intermediate, and parabasal.

#### 1.7.1.1 Superficial Squamous Cells

They are the most mature and consist of large, polygonal cells with abundant glassy cytoplasm. The cytoplasm can be pink, orange, or blue/green in Pap stain depending on the degree of maturation of the keratin granules. The nuclei are small, about 15–20 $\mu m^2$, and pyknotic, resembling an ink dot (Fig. 1.7).

#### 1.7.1.2 Intermediate Squamous Cells

They are similar to superficial cells, except that the nuclei are larger, about 35 $\mu m^2$, with open, finely granular chromatin (Fig. 1.7). The cytoplasm may appear yellow because of the presence of glycogen.

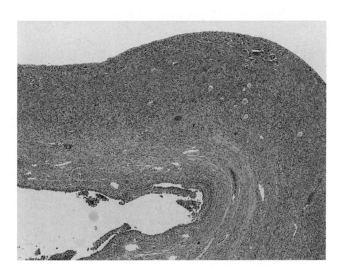

**Fig. 1.6** Normal ovarian cortex with follicles at various maturation stages (H.E. ×40)

**Fig. 1.7** Normal superficial
and intermediate squamous
cells. Both superficial and
intermediate squamous cells
are polygonal with abundant
translucent cytoplasm.
Superficial squamous cells
possess small and hyper-
chromatic nuclei (ink dot
nuclei), whereas intermediate
squamous cells have bigger
nuclei with more open
chromatin (SurePath,
Papanicolaou, ×400)

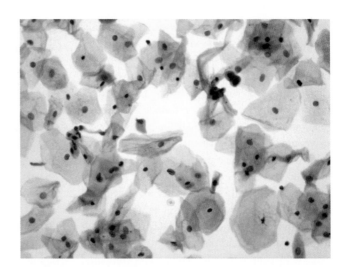

**Fig. 1.8** Normal parabasal
squamous cells. Parabasal
cells arrange either singly or
in two-dimensional groups.
Isolated parabasal cells are
round to oval with dense and
homogenous cytoplasm.
Parabasal cells in groups and
clusters may be difficult to
differentiate from metaplastic
squamous cells (SurePath,
Papanicolaou, ×400)

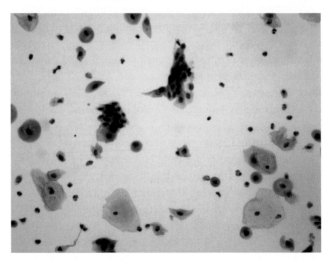

## 1.7.2 Parabasal Squamous Cells

They are the least mature and are usually identified only in women with immature epithelia due
to a lack of estrogenic stimulation such as that in
postmenopausal and postpartum women. The
parabasal cells are usually round to oval with
moderate amount of cyanophilic cytoplasm and
a larger (50 μm² in diameter) vesicular nucleus,
resulting in a higher N:C ratio. They can occur
singly, in groups, as large monolayer sheets, or
as syncytial aggregates. Preservation of nuclear
polarity and lack of nuclear pleomorphism distinguish normal parabasal cells from dysplastic
squamous cells (Fig. 1.8).

## 1.7.3 Endocervical Cells

Endocervical cells are usually present in sheets
with a honeycomb appearance, or in strip resembling a picket fence (Fig. 1.9). Single cells as well
as naked nuclei within strands of mucus can also
be seen. Individual cells appear columnar with
cyanophilic and clear cytoplasm. The nuclei are
round and basally located, similar to that of intermediate squamous cells. However, mild degree of
anisonucleosis may be evident.

The increasing use of brooms and brushes
coupled with liquid-based preparation (LBP)
yields large, densely packed groups of endocervical cells with significant nuclear overlapping

**Fig. 1.9** Normal endocervical cells. The endocervical cells arrange in either a two-dimensional sheet resembling a honeycomb or strips resembling a picket fence. Individual cells demonstrate well-defined cytoplasmic borders (SurePath, Papanicolaou, ×400)

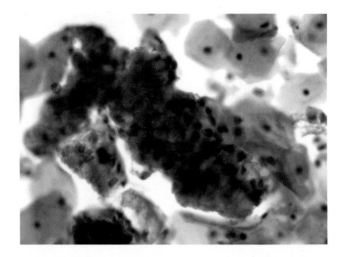

**Fig. 1.10** Large, three-dimensional group of endocervical cells commonly seen in LBP using brooms and brushes for collection (SurePath, Papanicolaou, ×100)

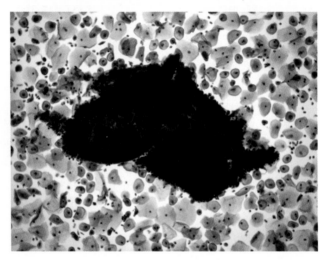

(Fig. 1.10). Individual cells can appear more hyperchromatic and demonstrate considerable degree of pleomorphism. Such changes may be misinterpreted as AEC. To avoid over interpretation, one should examine the periphery of the groups where normal-appearing endocervical cells are evident.

### 1.7.4 Squamous Metaplastic Cells

These are derived from the TZ where endocervical epithelium is gradually replaced by squamous epithelium. Mature squamous metaplastic cells are identical to intermediate and superficial squamous cells. Immature metaplastic cells

resemble parabasal cells and can occur singly, in small groups or chains, or in loose sheets. Cytoplasmic vacuoles and projections can be identified (Fig. 1.11).

### 1.7.5 Endometrial Cells

#### 1.7.5.1 Exfoliated Endometrial Glandular Cells

Normally, they can be observed up to 12 days after the last menstrual period (LMP). They often present as three-dimensional, tight clusters. Single cells are rare in conventional preparation but can be seen in LBP. Individual cells are small

**Fig. 1.11** Squamous metaplastic cells. Small cluster of metaplastic squamous cells appearing columnar or polygonal in shape. Cytoplasmic projections are frequently noted (SurePath, Papanicolaou, ×400)

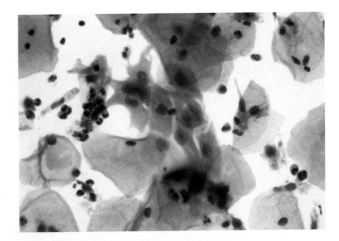

**Fig. 1.12** Exfoliated endometrial cells appearing as a tight cluster of small cells with scant cytoplasm (ThinPrep, Papanicolaou, ×400)

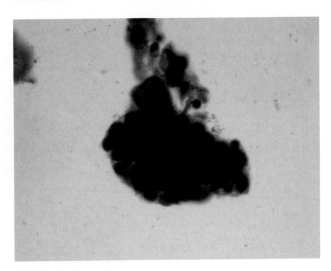

(35 μm²) with very scant amount of cytoplasm and indistinct cell borders. Occasional small cytoplasmic vacuoles can be seen. The nuclei are round to oval with darkly staining nuclei (Fig. 1.12). Tight groups of endometrial glandular cells surrounded by one or more layers of larger endometrial stromal cells with pale cytoplasm are termed exodus (Fig. 1.13). According to TBS 2001, only exfoliated endometrial cells should be reported in women aged 40 years or older.

### 1.7.5.2 Exfoliated Endometrial Stromal Cells

These cells often occur in loosely cohesive clusters. Individual cells possess cytanophilic, foamy cytoplasm and notched or bean-shaped nuclei, and are similar in size as the parabasal squamous cells. They may be mistaken for histiocytes (Fig. 1.14).

### 1.7.6 Direct Sampling of the Lower Uterine Segment

Vigorous sampling of the endocervical canal can result in the direct sampling of the lower uterine segment (LUS). The typical presentation is as large, complex, irregular tissue fragments with branching tubular glands, on low magnification (Fig. 1.15). Higher magnification often reveals a biphasic pattern of inner glandular cells and outer stromal cells (Fig. 1.16). The latter appears as bland, elongated to oval cells, often embedded in a small amount of matrix in a relatively disorderly pattern.

**Fig. 1.13** Exodus consisting of a central tight group of endometrial glandular cells surrounded by layers of larger, pale endometrial stromal cells (SurePath, Papanicolaou, ×400)

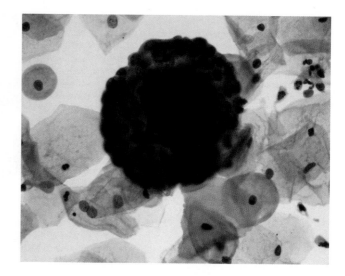

**Fig. 1.14** Cohesive group of endometrial stromal cells with round to oval degenerated nuclei and moderate amount of foamy cytoplasm (SurePath, Papanicolaou, ×400)

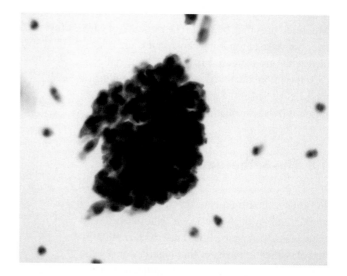

**Fig. 1.15** Lower uterine segment showing large tissue fragment with branching tubular glands (SurePath, Papanicolaou, ×100)

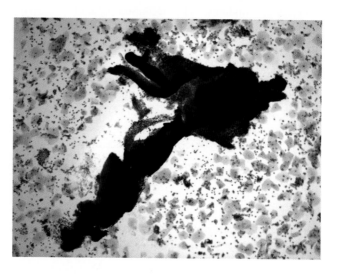

**Fig. 1.16** Higher magnification of lower uterine segment showing a biphasic pattern: endometrial cells (*upper right hand*) and stromal cells (*center*) (SurePath, Papanicolaou, ×400)

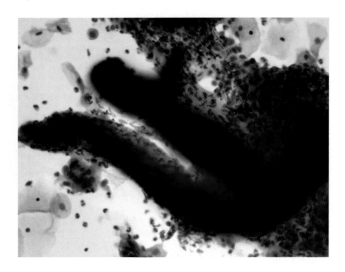

Mitotic figures may be seen. The presence of LUS does not warrant reporting because it is not associated with any increased risk of endometrial cancers. It is important to recognize direct sampling of the LUS because it is one of the differential diagnoses of hyperchromatic crowded groups.

## 1.8 The Bethesda System

In order to communicate the results effectively and unambiguously between laboratories and clinicians, cytologists should use the terminology and classification system that clearly convey the diagnostic interpretation and significance of the morphologic findings. The Bethesda system (TBS), first introduced in 1988, offers a model for the uniform descriptive terminology for reporting cervicovaginal cytology. The current TBS, which was adopted after an international consensus conference in 2001, is summarized in Table 1.1. The report format includes (1) specimen type, (2) specimen adequacy, (3) general categorization, and (4) descriptive interpretations, and is applicable to both conventional and liquid-based preparations.

Although TBS is widely in use throughout USA and much of the World, there are other systems of cervical cytology classification, such as those proposed by the British Society for

**Table 1.1** The Bethesda system 2001 for reporting cervicovaginal cytology

Specimen type
  Specify whether the preparation is conventional, ThinPrep, or SurePath
Specimen adequacy
  Satisfactory for evaluation
  Presence or absence of endocervical/transformation zone
  Other quality-limiting factors such as obscuring inflammation
  Unsatisfactory for evaluation
    Specify reasons
General categorization (optional)
  Negative for intraepithelial lesion or malignancy
  Epithelial cell abnormality (see below)
  Other
Descriptive interpretations
  Nonneoplastic
    Organisms
    *Trichomonas vaginalis*
    Fungal organisms consistent with *Candida* spp.
    Shift in bacterial flora suggestive of bacterial vaginosis
    Bacterial morphologically consistent with *Actinomyces* spp.
    Cellular changes associated with herpes simplex virus
      Other nonneoplastic findings
    Reactive cellular changes (including typical repairs)
    Radiation
    Atrophy
    Benign-appearing glandular cells status post-hysterectomy
  Other
    Endometrial cells in women over 40 years of age

(continued)

**Table 1.1** (continued)

Epithelial cell abnormalities
  Squamous cell
    Atypical squamous cells of undetermined
      significance (ASC-US)
    Atypical squamous cells cannot exclude HSIL (ASC-H)
    Low-grade squamous intraepithelial lesions (LSIL)
    High-grade squamous intraepithelial lesions (HSIL)
    Squamous cell carcinoma
  Glandular cell
    Atypical endocervical cells (AEC)
    Atypical glandular cells (AGC)
    Atypical endometrial cells (AMC)
    Atypical endocervical cells, favor neoplastic
    Atypical glandular cells, favor neoplastic
    Endocervical adenocarcinoma in situ (AIS)
    Adenocarcinoma (specify type if possible)
  Other malignant neoplasms (specify if possible)
Ancillary studies (optional)
Educational notes and recommendations (optional)

translatable into TBS. A comparison of TBS with the other terminology systems is included in Table 1.2.

## 1.8.1 Specimens Adequacy

TBS 2001 requires that a statement of the specimen adequacy be given in the report. There are two adequacy categories: satisfactory and unsatisfactory. The later can be due to insufficient squamous cellularity and/or obscuring factors. In addition, any specimen with abnormal cells is considered to be satisfactory.

Clinical Cytology (BSCC) and Australia National Pathology Accreditation Advisory Council. Although a unified classification system does not exist for all the members of the European Union, it is recommended that any systems should be

## 1.8.2 Minimum Squamous Cellularity Criteria

TBS 2001 requires at least 8,000–12,000 and 5,000 well-preserved and well-visualized squamous cells on a conventional smear and a LBP, respectively. For conventional preparation, instead of actually counting individual cells, the

**Table 1.2** Comparison of reporting systems for gynecologic cytology

| TBS 2001 | CIN | BSCC 2008 | ECTP 2007 | AMBS 2004 |
|---|---|---|---|---|
| NILM | | Negative | Within normal limits | Negative |
| Unsatisfactory | | Inadequate | Unsatisfactory | Unsatisfactory |
| ASC-US | | Borderline changes, squamous, NOS | Squamous cell changes (not definitively neoplastic but merit early repeat) | Possible LSIL |
| ASC-H | | Borderline changes, high-grade dyskaryosis not excluded | | Possible HSIL |
| LSIL | HPV cytopathic changes | Low-grade dyskaryosis | Koilocytes (w/o changes s/o SIL) | LSIL |
| | CIN I | | Mild dysplasia (CIN I) | |
| HSIL | CIN II | High-grade dyskaryosis | Moderate dysplasia (CIN II) | HSIL |
| | CIN III/CIS | | Severe dysplasia (CIN III) Carcinoma in situ | |
| SCC | SCC | SCC | SCC | SCC |
| AGC, AEC | | Borderline changes in endocervical cells | AGC | AGC, AEC |
| AIS | AIS | | | EC AIS |
| Adenocarcinoma | Adenocarcinoma | Glandular neoplasia | Adenocarcinoma | Adenocarcinoma |

**Fig. 1.17** Atrophy specimen showing parabasal squamous cells indistinguishable from metaplastic squamous cells (SurePath, Papanicolaou, ×100)

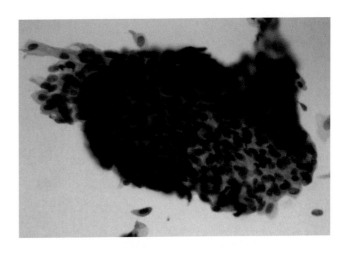

squamous cellularity should be estimated by comparing to computer-generated reference images to stimulate the appearance of 4× fields on conventional smears. For LBP, cellularity can be estimated by performing representative field cell counts. Based on the preparation diameter and the ocular eyepiece, one can estimate the average number of cells per field required to achieve a minimum of 5,000 cells.

### 1.8.3 Endocervical/Transformation Zone Component

TBS 2001 defines an adequate endocervical/transformation zone (EC/TZ) component as the presence of ten or more well-preserved endocervical and/or squamous metaplastic cells. This criterion applies to all pre- and postmenopausal women, except that in women with marked atrophy, parabasal squamous cells often cannot be distinguished from metaplastic and endocervical cells (Fig. 1.17). The lack of EC/TZ component, by itself, does not make a specimen unsatisfactory. Data regarding whether a lack of EC/TZ component correlates negatively with the detection of high-grade squamous lesions are conflicting.

### 1.8.4 Obscuring Factors

When more than 75% of squamous cells are obscured by factors such as inflammation, blood, and very thick smears, the specimen should be classified as unsatisfactory. Mild cytolysis is usually acceptable; however, if nearly all nuclei are naked, i.e., devoid of cytoplasm, the specimens should be classified as unsatisfactory. For LBP, the combination of some degree of obscuring factors and borderline squamous cellularity may render the specimen unsatisfactory because of a lack of sufficient number of well-visualized and well-preserved squamous cells.

### 1.8.5 Management of Women with Unsatisfactory Pap Test

According to the 2006 American Society of Colposcopy and Cervical Pathology (ASCCP) management guidelines for abnormal Pap tests, a repeat Pap test should be performed within a 2- to 4-month period for women with an unsatisfactory Pap tests. Women lacking EC/TZ component and/or other quality indicators, but with a negative Pap test should have a repeat Pap test in 12 months.

## Suggested Reading

Denton KJ, et al. The revised BSCC terminology for abnormal cervical cytology. Cytopathology. 2008;19: 137–57.

Diane S, Nayar R, Davey DD, and Wilbur DC. The Bethesda System for Reporting Cervical Cytology: Definitions, Criteria, and Explanatory Notes. 2nd Edn. Springer, Berlin. 2004

Herbert A, et al. European guidelines for quality assurance in cervical cancer screening: recommendations for cervical cytology terminology. Cytopathology. 2007;18:213–9.

Herzberg AJ, Raso DS, Silverman JF, and Allpress SM. Color Atlas of Normal Cytology. 1st Edn. Churchill Livingstone, New York. 1999.

Mills SE (2006). Histology for Pathologists. 3rd Edn. Raven Press, New York.

# Chapter 2
# Lesions of the Vulva and Vagina

**Keywords** Vulva • Vagina • Dysplasia • Carcinoma • Melanoma

with benign angiomyofibroblastoma and deep aggressive angiomyxoma primarily involving these areas.

## 2.1 General Classification of Tumors or Tumor-Like Conditions of Vulva and Vagina

Tumors of vulva and vagina are generally classified into squamous, glandular, melanocytic, and mesenchymal neoplasms. Squamous carcinoma is by far the most common primary malignancy involving both organs. Squamous intraepithelial neoplasia is the most common preinvasive condition of squamous cell carcinoma (SCC). Lichen sclerosus is also considered as a preneoplastic condition of vulvar SCC (Fig. 2.1). Condyloma acuminatum is the most common squamous disorder, caused by low-risk HPV subtypes (HPV 6 and 11), and does not progress to malignancy, except in rare cases where high-risk HPV is a causal factor. Conventional mullerian adenocarcinomas are rare in vulva and vagina. Extramammary Paget's disease represents a special form of glandular malignancy outside of the breast and is generally not associated with an invasive component. Primary clear cell carcinoma of the vagina is famous for its association with intrauterine DES exposure in the past, but is very rare nowadays. Melanoma represents 5% of vulvar cancers and is capable of widespread metastasis. A variety of benign and malignant mesenchymal tumors can be seen in the vulvar and vaginal regions,

## 2.2 Benign, Preneoplastic, and In Situ Neoplastic Squamous Lesions

*Squamous cell hyperplasia* of the vulva is a thickened plaque-like lesion consisting of maturing squamous proliferation with hyperkeratosis and/or parakeratosis. No cytologic atypia is present (Fig. 2.2). The diagnosis requires the exclusion of other squamous proliferative disorders, particularly a condyloma.

*Squamous papilloma* of the vulva may be multiple and consists of simple papillary proliferation of squamous epithelium without complex branching (Fig. 2.3). The absence of definite HPV koilocytosis distinguishes it from a condyloma.

*Seborrheic keratosis* involves hair-bearing squamous epithelium of the vulva. Multiple lesions may be associated with Leser–Trelat syndrome. The lesion is characterized by symmetric squamous acanthosis, papillomatosis, and hyperkeratosis with keratin horn cysts (Fig. 2.4). Cytologic atypia and HPV-related koilocytosis are absent.

*Condyloma acuminatum* is a common, sexually transmitted, papillomatous squamous proliferation related to HVP 6 and 11, and is not

D. Chhieng and P. Hui (eds.), *Cytology and Surgical Pathology of Gynecologic Neoplasms*, Current Clinical Pathology, DOI 10.1007/978-1-60761-164-6_2, © Springer Science+Business Media, LLC 2011

**Fig. 2.1** Vulvar lichen sclerosus. Note the blunting of the rete pegs and the presence of homogenous collagen deposition in the upper dermis (H.E. ×40)

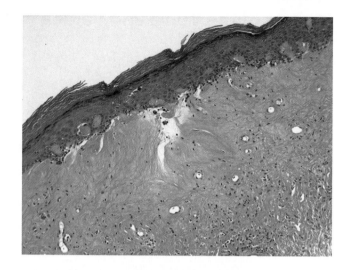

**Fig. 2.2** Vulvar squamous hyperplasia. Note the presence of acanthosis and hyperkeratosis, and the absence of HPV-related koilocytosis and epithelial cell dysplasia (H.E. ×200)

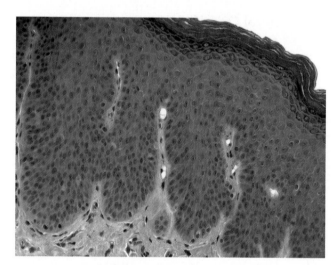

**Fig. 2.3** Vulvar squamous papilloma. Note the papillo-matosis and the absence of HPV-related koilocytopathic effect (H.E. ×40)

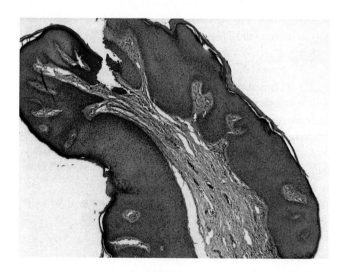

**Fig. 2.4** Seborrheic keratosis. Note the symmetric squamous acanthosis, papillomatosis, and hyperkeratosis with keratin horn cysts (H.E. ×40)

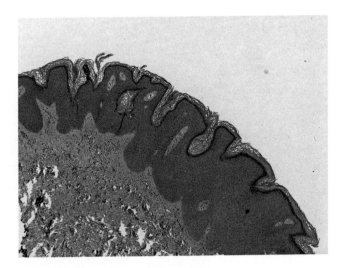

considered progressive toward invasive cancer. Its appearance is clinically distinct with a verrucous growth and is frequently multifocal, and even confluent, involving large areas. Histologically, the lesion consists of papillomatous squamous proliferation with fibrous stroma (Fig. 2.5a). Marked acanthosis, parakeratois, and hyperkeratosis are common. The hallmark of condyloma is the presence of koilocytes. Koilocytosis frequently involves superficial areas of the lesion with nuclear enlargement, multinucleation, hyperchromasia, irregular or raisinoid nuclear membrane, and perinuclear halo (Fig. 2.5b). Koilocytosis may be focal and involves clusters of superficial squamous cells. Prominent granulocytic layer is also characteristic. Distinguishing from a squamous papilloma requires the presence of koilocytes, and when in doubt, the presence of Ki-67 positive nuclei in the upper half of the epithelium favors a diagnosis of condyloma.

*Squamous intraepithelial neoplasia* of vulva (VIN) or vagina (VAIN) is, by analogy to cervical intraepithelial lesions, divided into grades 1, 2, and 3, based on the presence of neoplastic/dysplastic squamous cells limited to the lower one-third, middle one-third, or the full thickness of the epithelium, respectively. The lesions clinically present as erythematous patches, or verruciform or even pigmented plaques. They may be multiple and involve large areas including the perineum. VIN and VAIN can be subclassified into (1) the so-called warty type when koilocytes are present, (2) bowenoid type when the lesion consists of smaller, basaloid yet cellular dysplastic cells without koilocytosis (Fig. 2.6), and (3) "differentiated" or simplex type, in which deceptive benign squamous papillomatosis is seen in association with paradoxical parakeratosis (cytoplasmic eosinophilia) in the lower half of the epithelium and dysplastic cells are limited to the basal layer. P53 immunostain may show a diffuse nuclear positivity throughout the entire epithelium.

*Invasive squamous cell carcinoma* is most commonly seen in patients over 60 years of age and may be proceeded by VIN or VAIN. Most well-differentiated SCCs (Fig. 2.7) arise from a background of dermatosis or lichen sclerosus, however. Warty and basaloid carcinomas can occur along with their corresponding intraepithelial neoplasia (Figs. 2.8 and 2.9). The well-differentiated verrucous carcinoma shows no significant cytologic atypia and obvious stromal invasion. The diagnosis can be extremely difficult and relies on the overall pushing growth pattern into the underlying stroma (Fig. 2.10), usually requiring large, well-oriented excision or vulvectomy for its separation from condyloma, squamous papilloma, and pseudoepitheliomatous hyperplasia. Poorly differentiated SCCs are not uncommon in vulva and vagina. Anaplastic, acantholytic,

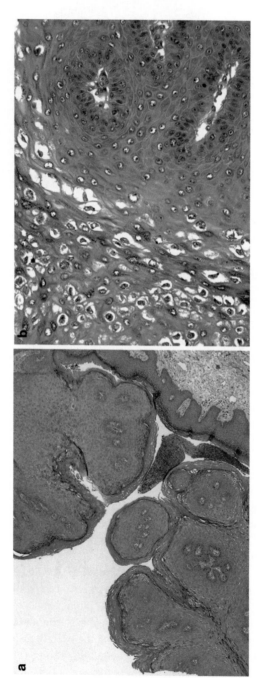

**Fig. 2.5** Condyloma acuminatum. Note the marked papillomatosis, acanthosis, parakeratosis, and hyperkeratosis (**a**) (H.E. ×40). The hallmark of condyloma is the presence of koilocytes (**b**) (H.E. ×200)

**Fig. 2.6** Vulvar intraepithelial
neoplasia 2 (H.E. ×100)

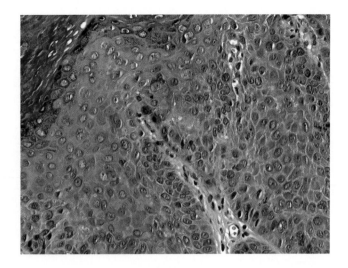

**Fig. 2.7** Vulvar well-
differentiated keratinizing
squamous cell carcinoma
(H.E. ×40)

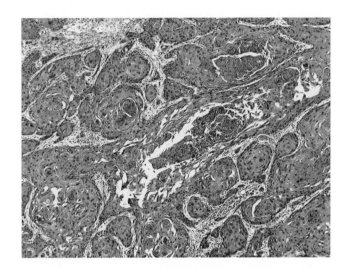

**Fig. 2.8** Warty squamous
cell carcinoma. Note the
condylomatous and
koilocytoid carcinomatous
nests (H.E. ×40)

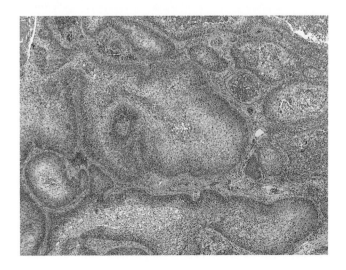

**Fig. 2.9** Basaloid squamous cell carcinoma of the vulva. Note the hypercellularity and palisading of tumor cells at the periphery of the tumor nests (H.E. ×40)

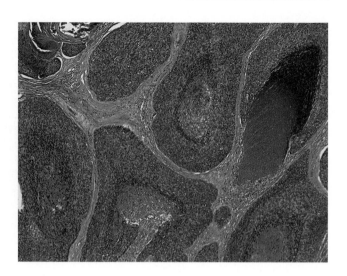

sarcomatoid, and lymphoepithelioma-like carcinomas are rare variants of SCC.

*Microinvasive squamous cell carcinoma* is diagnosed when early stromal invasion is less than 1 mm in depth. Its differential diagnosis from VIN or VAIN can be often difficult. Singles or irregular clusters of dysplastic epithelial cells extruding from the base of an in situ lesion are diagnostic. Isolated tumor nests with paradoxical maturation and haphazard arrangements of tumor cells are highly suggestive of early invasion (Fig. 2.11). A stromal response is almost always present, including desmoplasia, edema, and/or lymphoplasmacytic infiltration.

## 2.3 Glandular Lesions

### 2.3.1 Benign Glandular Lesions

Common tumor-like conditions include epidermal inclusion cyst, Bartholin cyst (location is important for diagnosis, Fig. 2.12), Bartholin gland hyperplasia (Fig. 2.13), mucinous cyst and ciliated cyst, ectopic breast tissue with associated benign conditions (adenosis and papilloma), and others. *Hidradenoma* (papilliferum or clear cell) is the most common vulvar benign glandular tumor. It is usually asymptomatic and small (less than 1 cm), frequently involving the labia majora. Majority of cases of hidradenoma papilliferum are nodular and composed of compact glandular or tubular epithelial growth with papillary formations. The epithelium is, at least focally, double layered with inner tall columnar glandular cells and outer myoepithelial cells (Fig. 2.14a, b). The lobulated clear cell variant is solid and consists of tumor cells with clear cytoplasm and uniform nuclei (Fig. 2.15). The presence of hyalinized stroma is frequently found. The absence of infiltrative border and minimal cytologic atypia attest the benignancy of both subtypes of hidradenoma. The presence of mitosis in both variants, even frequent, does not necessarily indicate malignancy. Benign mixed tumor is essentially similar to that of the salivary glands. Vaginal benign glandular tumor or tumor-like lesions are less frequent and include DES-related adenosis (mucinous, tuboendometrial, and embryonic types), microglandular hyperplasia, and Mullerian papilloma of infancy.

### 2.3.2 Adenocarcinomas

Adenocarcinomas of the vulva and the vagina are rare, among which vulvar Paget's disease and vaginal clear cell carcinomas are of special concern.

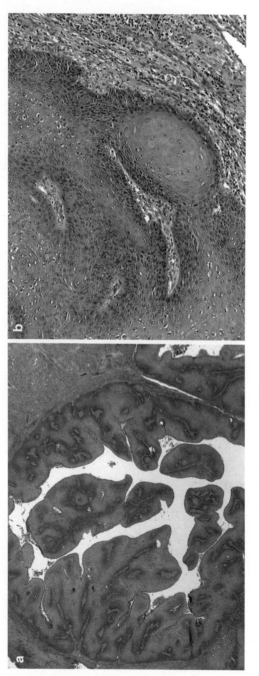

**Fig. 2.10** (**a**, **b**) Verrucous squamous carcinoma. Note the deceptive well-differentiated squamous epithelium and the pushing invasion into the underlying stroma (H.E. ×20 (**a**), ×100 (**b**))

**Fig. 2.11** Microinvasive squamous cell carcinoma. Note the isolated tumor nests with paradoxical maturation and haphazard arrangements of tumor cells (H.E. ×40)

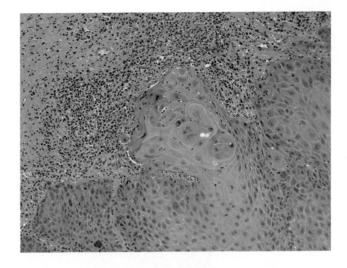

**Fig. 2.12** Bartholin gland cyst. Note the presence of Bartholin gland hyperplasia (H.E. ×100)

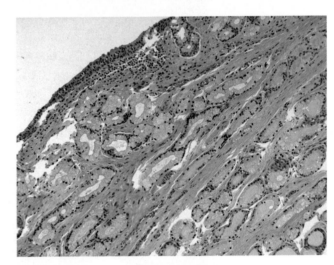

**Fig. 2.13** Bartholin gland hyperplasia. Note the lobular hyperplasia of mucinous glands (H.E. ×40)

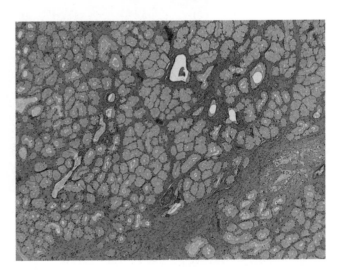

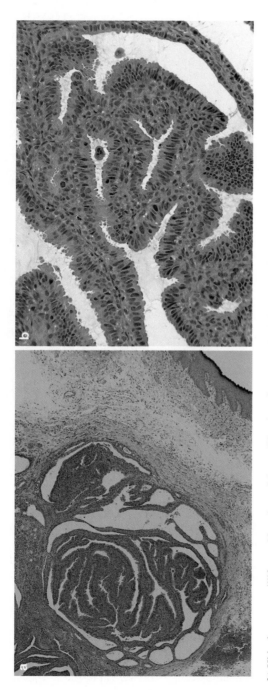

**Fig. 2.14** (**a**, **b**) Hidradenoma papilliferum. Note the nodular proliferation of compact glandular or tubular epithelial growth with papillary formations (**a**, H.E, ×40), and the presence of double layers of inner tall columnar glandular cells and outer myoepithelial cells (**b**, H.E, ×200)

**Fig. 2.15** Clear cell
hidradenoma. The tumor
consists of lobules of solid
tumor cells with clear
cytoplasm and uniform nuclei
(H.E. ×40)

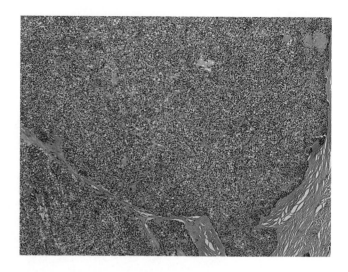

**Fig. 2.16** Vulvar Paget's
disease. Note the presence of
scattered single or clusters
of large mucin-containing
cells involving the lower half
of the squamous epithelium
(H.E. ×200)

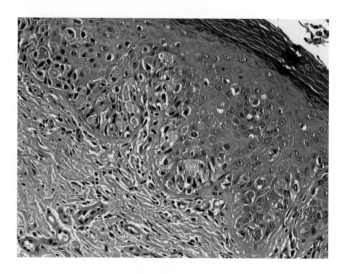

*Vulvar Paget's disease* is a form of in situ adenocarcinoma of the extramammary Toker-like cell. It represents 5% of vulvar malignancy. Characteristically, the tumor demonstrates as red eczematous plaques in the agnogenital region of an older Caucasian woman. Her-2/neu protein overexpression and/or gene amplification are frequently seen (up to 50%). Histologically, the involved epidermis is disrupted by scattered single or clusters of large mucin-containing cells involving the lower half or entire epithelium. The tumor cells have abundant pale cytoplasm with central round nuclei (Fig. 2.16). Mitosis can be frequent. They may replace the entire epithelium or spread into hair follicles or other skin adnexal structures. However, invasive vulvar Paget's disease is rare. The main differential diagnoses include malignant melanoma and colonization of the vulva by urothelial or anal carcinomas. Paget cells are characteristically stained for mucin (PAS, Alcian blue, and mucicarmine) and CAM5.2, CK7, GCDFP, MUDC5AC, and CEA, in contrast to melanocytic markers (HMB45 and Mel-A) expressed in melanomas. The presence of glandular structure within the tumor nests is highly suggestive of Paget's disease. Patients with Pagetoid spreading of an anal-rectal adenocarcinoma usually have a documented history and the tumor cells are positive for CK20 but negative for CK7. Spreading of an urothelial carcinoma to the vulva likely demonstrates an immunohistochemical profile of CK7 and CK20 positivity and GCDFP negativity.

*Vaginal clear cell carcinoma* has become very rare as the population with possible DES exposure is in their postmenopausal age. The tumor typically occurs in adolescents and young adults with average age at diagnosis of 17 years. Vaginal bleeding or discharge is typical clinical presentation. Vaginal adenosis, cervical ectropion, or transverse septum or cervical ridges are commonly associated with clear cell carcinoma of the vagina. Most tumors are superficially invasive at presentation. Three major histologic growth patterns are seen: tubulocystic, sold, and papillary. The most common tubulocystic variant consists of round to oval cystic glands or tubules lined by flat, cuboidal, or columnar cells with abundant clear cytoplasm. Marked cytologic atypia and frequent mitotic activities are present in most tumors. Characteristically, hobnailing of the marked atypical cells can be found, at least focally (Fig. 2.17). Extracellular mucin production may be seen, whereas intracellular mucin production is extremely rare. The papillary variant consists of glands or cysts lined by hierarchical papillary proliferation of clear cells. Psammoma bodies may occasionally be seen. In the solid type, the tumor cells are polygonal with abundant glycogenated clear cytoplasm and sharp demarcated borders (simulating vegetable cells), and grow in solid sheets.

## 2.4 Other Epithelial or Epithelioid Lesions

*Carcinomas of the Bartholin gland* represent 5% of vulvar cancers with diagnostic qualifiers including tumor involving Bartholin gland area, histologic transition between normal and carcinoma components, and no primary tumor elsewhere. Histologic variants of Bartholin gland carcinomas include squamous cell carcinoma (40%), adenocarcinoma (25%), adenocystic carcinoma (12%), and other types (mucinous of the intestinal type, adenosquamous, transitional cell, and undifferentiated including small cell neuroendocrine carcinomas). Of the patients with Bartholin gland carcinomas, 40% present with nodal metastasis. The overall 10-year survival is 60%.

*Adenocarcinoma of the mammary type* is rare and likely arises from the ectopic breast tissue. These tumors resemble conventional breast ductal and lobular carcinomas. Metastatic breast lesions must be ruled out before such diagnosis is made.

*Basal cell carcinomas* account for 3% of vulvar cancers, and are typically seen in elderly

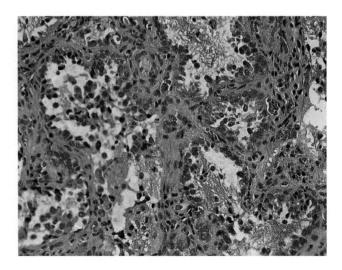

**Fig. 2.17** Vaginal clear cell carcinoma. Note the tubulocystic spaces lined by flat, cuboidal, or columnar cells with abundant clear cytoplasm. Marked cytologic atypia and frequent mitotic activities are present. (H.E. ×200)

patients and frequently with extravulvar basal cell carcinoma.

*Vaginal primary yolk sac tumor* affects children less than 3 years of age and accounts for 90% of extragonadal yolk sac tumor. Vaginal polypoid lesion with bleeding is common and AFP is typically elevated at presentation. The histologic features are similar to those of the gonadal counterpart with reticular growth patterns, the presence of Schiller–Duval bodies and eosinophilic globular bodies. A cure can be achieved by combined chemotherapy with or without surgery in most cases.

## 2.5 Melanocytic Lesions

Malignancy melanoma represents 5–10% of vulvar or vaginal cancers, typically seen in elderly patients with atypical extravulvar melanocytic lesions. Pigmented irregular plaques or nodules are seen in most cases, although amelanotic melanoma is not uncommon. The majority of the cases are of mucosal lentiginous type with spindle invasive cells and prominent perineural invasion. The main differential diagnoses include vulvar Paget's disease (see above) and poorly differentiated carcinomas.

## 2.6 Mesenchymal and Lymphoid Neoplasms

Although rare, a variety of benign and malignant soft tissue tumors involve vulva and vagina. Relatively common benign soft tissue tumors or tumor-like lesions include fibroepithelial polyp, angiomyofibroblastoma, postoperative spindle cell nodule, nodular fasciitis, dermatofibroma, leiomyoma, rhabdomyoma, granular cell tumor (Fig. 2.18), and others. Aggressive angiomyoma, leiomyosarcoma, proximal epithelioid sarcoma, rhabdomyosarcoma, and others are among malignant soft tissue tumors. Diffuse large B-cell lymphoma is the most common lymphoproliferative disorder.

*Fibroepithelial polyp* is a common polypoid lesion covered by simple, mature squamous epithelium (Fig. 2.19a). Frequently, the stromal myofibroblasts are multinucleated and bizarre in appearance. A cellular pseudosarcomatous fibroepithelial polyp may show hypercellular stromal cells with marked pleomorphism, nuclear hyperchromatia, mitotic activity of more than 10 mitosis/10 high-power fields (HPF), and even atypical mitoses (Fig. 2.19b).

*Postoperative spindle cell nodule* is a polypoid or nodular reactive spindle cell proliferation that develops a few months after hysterectomy.

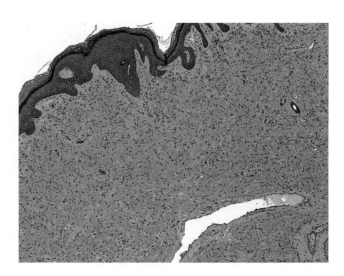

**Fig. 2.18** Vulvar granular cell tumor (H.E. ×100)

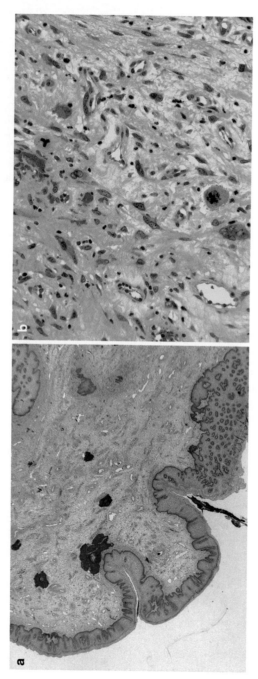

**Fig. 2.19** (**a, b**) Vaginal fibroepithelial polyp. Pseudosarcomatous stroma is present in the particular vaginal polyp (H.E. ×40 (**a**), ×200 (**b**))

**Fig. 2.20** Angiomyofibroblastoma of the vulva. Note
the nodules of alternating
cellular to hypocellular
proliferations of small round
to spindle cells with
eosinophilic cytoplasm,
embedded in an edematous to
collagenous matrix.
Hemangiopericytoma-like
vasculature is present
(H.E. ×40)

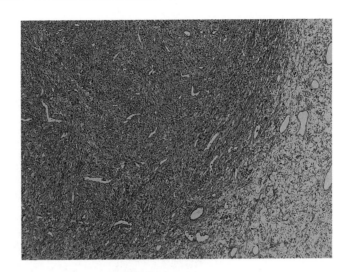

The lesion consists of fascicles of spindle myofibroblasts in a background of delicate capillaries and inflammatory cells. Mitoses are numerous.

*Angiomyofibroblastoma* involves almost exclusively vulvovaginal soft tissue. Usually, the lesion is less than 5 cm in size with a sharply defined margin. Histologically, the tumor consists of alternating cellular to hypocellular proliferations of small, round to spindle cells with eosinophilic cytoplasm, embedded in an edematous to collagenous matrix. Somewhat epithelioid tumor cells are typically clustered around capillaries (Fig. 2.20). The spindle cells are immunoreactive for desmin.

*Aggressive angiomyxoma* is a locally recurrent, deep-seated, soft tissue tumor involving mainly pelvicoperineal soft tissue of women in their reproductive age. The tumor is often more than 10 cm in size and poorly circumscribed. The lesion is grossly gelatinous and imperceptively infiltrates into adjacent structures. Histologically, the tumor is usually hypocellular with abundant edematous to myxoid matrix (Fig. 2.21a). The tumor consists of uniformly bland, short spindle cells with round nuclei and eosinophilic cytoplasm with cytoplasmic processes. Clusters of vasculatures of various calibers, including medium to large arterials, are characteristically present, and some of the vessels may be cuffed by eosinophilic collagen (Fig. 2.21b). The tumor cells are reactive for desmin, SMA, ER, and PR. The deep location, infiltrative margin, uniform

paucicellularity, and typical vascular clustering with collagen cuffing separate the tumor from superficial angiomyxoma, angiomyofibroblastoma, and fibroepithelial polyp. Adequate resection with generous margins cures most of the tumor without further recurrence.

*Leiomyoma and leiomyosarcoma* of vulva and vagina are rare smooth muscle tumors. Leiomyomas are much more common than leiomyosarcomas. Most leiomyomas are conventional mature smooth muscle tumors (Fig. 2.22). Epithelioid and myxoid leiomyomas can also occur. A diagnosis of malignancy follows the criteria similar to those of a soft tissue leiomyosarcoma, including the presence of two of the following: tumor more than 5 cm in size, more than 2–5 mitotic figures per 10 HPF, and moderate or severe cytologic atypia.

*Botryoid rhabdomyosarcoma* (sarcoma botryoides) is a rare sarcoma of patients under 5 years of age. Polypoid or lobulated tumor with myxoid stroma containing primitive round to spindle cells are characteristic. The presence of cambium layer (condensed tumor cells underneath the tumor surface) and the finding of rhabdomyoblasts are diagnostic clues.

*Proximal epithelioid sarcoma* involves principally the genital area, with more aggressive behavior than those of the distal counterpart. A multinodular growth with large eosinophilic, epithelioid tumor cells is characteristic (Fig. 2.23). The tumor cells are strongly reactive for cytokeratin, EMA, and CD34 immunohistochemistry.

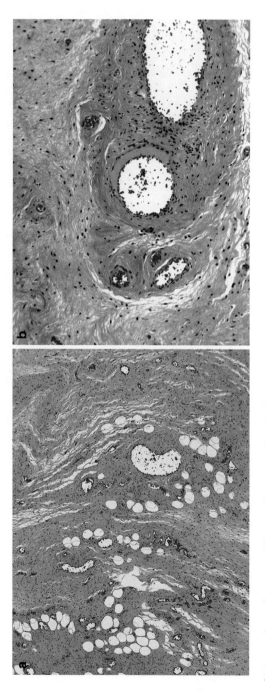

**Fig. 2.21** (**a, b**) Aggressive angiomyxoma. The tumor is hypocellular with abundant edematous to myxoid matrix with invasion into adjacent adipose tissue (**a**, H.E. ×40). Clusters of vasculatures of various calibers, including medium to large arterials, are characteristically present, and some of the vessels may be cuffed by eosinophilic collagen (**b**, H.E. ×100)

**Fig. 2.22** Vulvar leiomyoma
(H.E. ×40)

**Fig. 2.23** Proximal
epithelioid sarcoma. Note the
nodular growth with large
eosinophilic, epithelioid
tumor cells and vague
granulomatous configuration
(H.E. ×40)

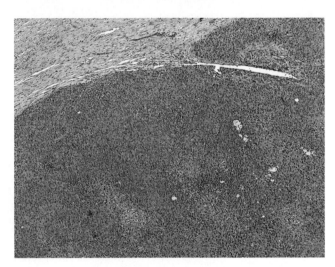

Expression of desmin and SMA can also been demonstrated. The differential diagnoses include poorly differentiate carcinomas and melanoma, which can be resolved by typical immunohistochemical phenotypes of each tumors. The presence of in situ melanocytic lesion favors malignant melanoma.

*Vulvar and vaginal lymphomas* are mostly secondary. Primary lymphomas account for roughly one-third. Although there is a wide range of histologic subtypes, diffuse large B-cell lymphoma is the single most common subtype. Misdiagnosis of vulvar and vaginal lymphomas is common and a diagnosis of "lymphoma-like lesion" should be used with caution. Consultation

with a hematopathologist should be made when in doubt.

## 2.7 Secondary Tumors

Secondary tumors of the vagina are at least four times more common than primary lesions. Most are direct extension from a cervical or an endometrial cancer (50%). Metastatic tumors from breast, colorectum, ovary, and even left kidney can occur. Similar metastatic tumor types can involve the vulva, half of which are gynecologic primaries.

## 2.8  Cytology of Vulva

For nonulcerated lesions, vigorous scraping of the area with sampling devices such as the scalpel blade or spatula is necessary for obtaining cellular materials which can then be smeared on the slides. Placing a warm, moist towel or cloth over the lesion helps softens the superficial keratinizing layers and increases the cellular yield. For ulcerated lesions, sampling can be achieved by swabbing the edge of the ulcer or directly touching the lesion with a glass slide. The slides should be fixed immediately by immersing in 95% ethanol or using a spray fixative. Pigmented lesions should be best sampled by biopsy.

### 2.8.1  Dysplasia (Vulvar Intraepithelial Neoplasia)

Similar to their cervical counterpart, a two-tier classification system is used in vulvar cytology; low-grade vulvar lesions encompass VIN 1 and HPV cytopathic changes and high-grade vulvar lesions encompass VIN 2 and 3. Although the cytologic findings are similar to those of their cervical counterparts, hyperkeratosis and perarkeratosis are frequent and often obscure any rare dysplastic cells that may be present. This may explain a recent report of a lack of correlation between vulvar cytologic findings and histologic degree of VIN.

### 2.8.2  Squamous Cell Carcinoma

For most instances, the cytologic findings of vulvar SCC are similar to those of their cervical counterparts. However, there are a few variants that deserve special attention. Verrucous carcinoma is characterized by sheets of anucleated and parakeratotic squamous cells. Nuclear atypia is often minimal; therefore, a definitive cytologic diagnosis of malignancy is often impossible. Basal cell carcinoma presents with small and uniform neoplastic cells with scant cytoplasm and hyperchromatic nucleoli.

### 2.8.3  Paget's Disease

The neoplastic cells are large with a variable amount of cytoplasm, large eccentrically placed nuclei, and prominent nucleoli. Occasional large cytoplasmic vacuoles or signet ring-like cells can be seen. The cells arrange either singly or in small groups. Cells-in-cells arrangement is thought to be typical of Paget's disease. The differential diagnosis includes nonkeratinizing SCC and malignant melanoma. Biopsy and ancillary studies are necessary to arrive at the right diagnosis.

### 2.8.4  Mimics of Neoplastic Diseases

Pemphigus vulgaris is a noninfectious inflammatory disease that may sometimes involve the vulva. Diagnostic material can be obtained by scraping the base of the lesion and consists of isolated and loosely cohesive aggregates of acantholytic squamous cells. The latter is characterized by round to oval, large nuclei with vesicular chromatin and prominent nucleoli and may be mistaken as malignant cells (Fig. 2.24). Biopsy and immunofluorescence studies are required for a definitive diagnosis.

Lichen sclerosis and other dermatoses characterized by squamous cell hyperplasia demonstrate similar cytologic findings, showing a mixture of nucleated and anucleated squamous cells as well as parakeratotic squamous cells (Fig. 2.25). Reactive atypia may be evident and should not be confused with dysplastic changes.

## 2.9  Cytology of Vagina

Collection methods for exfoliative vaginal cytology are similar to those for cervical cytology. To avoid contamination, vaginal cytology samples should be obtained before sampling the cervix.

**Fig. 2.24** Pemphigus
vulgaris. Loosely cohesive
groups of squamous cells
with large, round nuclei and
prominent nucleoli
(conventional preparation,
Papanicolaou, ×400)

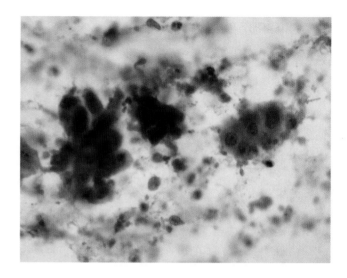

**Fig. 2.25** Lichen sclerosis.
Predominantly anucleated
squamous cells consistent
with hyperkeratosis.
(ThinPrep, Papanicolaou,
×400)

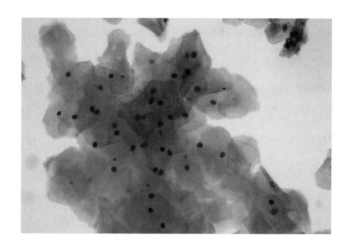

## 2.9.1 Diethylstilbestrol-Related Abnormalities

The incidence of DES-related vaginal adenosis
varies widely. Cytologically, the glandular cells
of vaginal adenosis resemble endocervical cells
with or without accompanying metaplastic
squamous cells. The tumor cells derived from
DES-related clear cell adenocarcinoma appear
singly or in small aggregates. Individual cells
have finely vacuolated cytoplasm, enlarged nuclei,
and macronucleoli. There is little variation in
nuclear size and shape.

## 2.9.2 Vaginal Intraepithelial Neoplasia

TBS is used for reporting vaginal cytology;
LSIL encompasses VAIN 1 and HPV cytopathic
changes and HSIL encompasses VAIN 2 and 3.
The cytologic findings are similar to those of
their cervical counterparts (Fig. 2.26). For most
patients with an abnormal Pap test and a cervix
in situ, the lesion is usually confined to the cervix. Occasionally, the dysplasia may extend
from the cervix to the vagina. In very rare
instances, when colposcopic examination and

**Fig. 2.26** Vaginal intraepithelial neoplasia III (VAIN III). Parabasal squamous cells with high N:C ratio, nuclear enlargement, and hyperchromasia (conventional preparation, Papanicolaou, ×400)

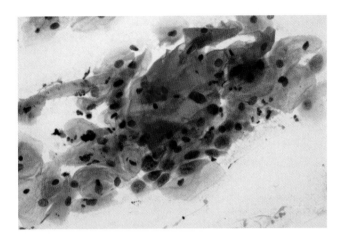

biopsy fail to identify any lesion in the cervix in the presence of a positive cervical cytology, the vagina should be carefully examined to rule out any VAIN.

### 2.9.3 Squamous Cell Carcinoma

Cytologically, SCC of the vagina cannot be distinguished from those that arise from other parts of the female genital tract.

### 2.9.4 Embryonal Rhabdomyosarcoma

The typical presentation is the finding of isolated and cohesive aggregates of small cells with eccentrically located, round to oval or elongated nuclei and a variable amount of cytoplasm. Tail-liked or broad band-like cytoplasmic projections are frequently present. The clinical presentation is also helpful; most patients are usually aged 5 years or younger and present with a grape-like mass expanding the vagina.

### 2.9.5 Mimics of Neoplastic Diseases

Atrophic vaginitis may be noted in postmenopausal women and other women who lack estrogen stimulation. Cytology of atrophic vaginitis has been previously described. Microorganisms such as candida, trichomonas, and bacteria can be seen in vaginal samples. The finding of benign glandular cells in vaginal cytology samples in patient status post-hysterectomy is of little clinical significance and not indicative of adenocarcinoma; this also applies to patients with a history of uterine adenocarcinoma.

### 2.9.6 Role of Vaginal Cytology Screening After Total Hysterectomy

Until recently, routine annual Pap test has been the standard practice for women who have had a hysterectomy for both benign and neoplastic diseases. However, this practice has come under discussion. Although patients with hysterectomy for benign conditions can occasionally develop primary vaginal neoplasia, it may not be cost effective to offer screening to these patients because of the very low incidence of primary vaginal neoplasia. Even for patients who had undergone hysterectomy for malignant diseases such as uterine endometrial adenocarcinoma, the incidence of asymptomatic vaginal recurrence of uterine cancer is less than 1%. Therefore, current guidelines suggest reducing or eliminating routine annual Pap test surveillance for patient status post-hysterectomy for both benign and malignant conditions. For symptomatic patients, appropriate examination and testing procedures should be performed promptly.

## Suggested Reading

Cooper AL, Dornfeld-Finke JM, Banks HW, Davey DD, Modesitt SC. Is cytologic screening an effective surveillance method for detection of vaginal recurrence of uterine cancer? Obstet Gynecol. 2006;107:71–6.

EJ Wilkinson. Premalignant and malignant tumors of the vulva. In Kurman RJ, ed. Blaustein's Pathology of the Female Genital Tract. 5th Edition. Springer, Berlin. 2002.

# Chapter 3
# Squamous Lesions of the Cervix

**Keywords** Cervix • Squamous intraepithelial lesion • Cervical intraepithelial lesion • Carcinoma

## 3.1 General Classification of Tumors of Cervix

Many neoplastic and preneoplastic lesions of the cervix are related to human papillomavirus (HPV) infection, particularly the high-risk subtypes. Squamous papillomas are benign proliferation of squamous epithelium and are related to low-risk HPV subtypes. Condyloma acuminatum is a manifestation of HPV infection, mostly in low-risk groups (HPV 6 and 11). Cervical intraepithelial neoplasia (CIN) 1 can harbor both the high- and low-risk subtypes of HPV. High-grade CIN (CIN 2 and 3) and invasive squamous cell carcinoma (SCC) are caused by high-risk HPV (HPV 16 and 18) and are associated with integrated viral genome. Primary adenocarcinomas of the cervix are associated with high-risk HPV infection in most, if not all, cases. The histologic spectrum of cervical adenocarcinomas includes usual endocervical adenocarcinoma, endometrioid carcinoma, and intestinal mucinous carcinoma, each of them may be accompanied by their corresponding in situ lesions. Rare variants include minimal deviation adenocarcinoma (adenoma malignum), villoglandular adenocarcinoma, adenosquamous carcinoma, adenobasal cell carcinoma, serous carcinoma, clear cell carcinoma, and neuroendocrine carcinomas.

## 3.2 Squamous Intraepithelial Lesions and Other HPV-Related Lesions

The spectrum of HPV-induced squamous lesions ranges from flat condyloma to invasive SCC. Flat condyloma, as its name indicates, is a plaque lesion involving ectocervix and transformation zone, with koilocytosis as the cardinal finding (Fig. 3.1). The koilocytic changes are recognized by cytoplasmic vacuolation around the nuclei with condensation of the cytoplasm at the periphery, nuclear atypicality including nuclear enlargement, hyperchromasia, chromatin clumping, and marked nuclear membrane irregularities, and multinucleation. Condyloma may coexist with low- (Fig. 3.2) or even high-grade CIN.

Low-grade CIN (CIN 1) should be separated from a pure condyloma. Parabasal cell proliferation with cytologic atypia is required for this separation (Fig. 3.2). The upper two-thirds of the epithelium show normal maturation and the dysplastic changes are limited to the lower third of the epithelium, including parabasal cell proliferation, nuclear enlargement, hyperchromasia, size variation, thickening of the nuclear membrane, and mitosis. The presence of mitotic figures several cell layers above the basal membrane supports a diagnosis of CIN 1. The presence of atypical mitosis even at the basal level also attests the presence of dysplasia, which some investigators consider as evidence of high-grade dysplasia. The upper two-thirds epithelium

D. Chhieng and P. Hui (eds.), *Cytology and Surgical Pathology of Gynecologic Neoplasms*, Current Clinical Pathology, DOI 10.1007/978-1-60761-164-6_3, © Springer Science+Business Media, LLC 2011

**Fig. 3.1** Cervical flat condyloma. Note the cytoplasmic vacuolation around the nuclei with condensation of the cytoplasm at the periphery, nuclear atypicality, and multinucleation (H.E. ×200)

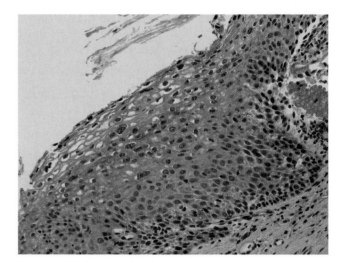

**Fig. 3.2** Cervical intraepithelial neoplasia 1 (CIN 1). Note the presence of atypical neoplastic proliferation limited to the lower third of the squamous epithelium (H.E. ×200)

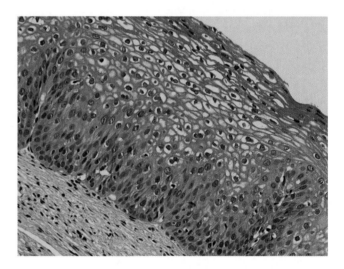

may show changes of HPV infection, although subtle in some cases.

CIN 2 is diagnosed when the neoplastic proliferation involves the lower and middle third of the epithelium, often with more pronounced cytologic atypia. Mitosis and atypical mitosis are easily identified. Loss of cell polarity, marked nuclear megaly, polymorphism, coarse chromatin condensation, large nucleolus, and atypical mitosis are frequently present (Fig. 3.3). It should be noted that a diagnosis of CIN 2 can be subjective and the least reproducible among CINs, yet its separation from CIN 1 is clinically relevant.

CIN 3 has minimal epithelial maturation and dysplastic cells involving all levels of the epithelium, frequently with numerous mitosis and atypical mitosis (Fig. 3.4).

Differential diagnosis of CINs can be difficult and subjective in some cases. Reactive squamous atypia, basal cell hyperplasia, squamous and atypical squamous metaplasia (Fig. 3.5), atrophy/transitional metaplasia (Fig. 3.6), lymphoid germinal center (Fig. 3.7), and tissue processing artifacts are frequently encountered situations. While their separation from a low-grade CIN may not be consequential, over-interpretation of these reactive

**Fig. 3.3**  Cervical intraepithelial neoplasia 2 (CIN 2) (H.E. ×200)

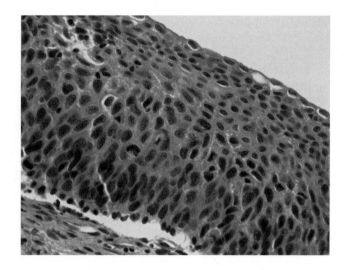

**Fig. 3.4**  Cervical intraepithelial neoplasia 3 (CIN 3) (H.E. ×100)

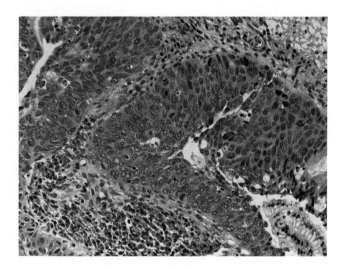

**Fig. 3.5**  Squamous metaplasia at the cervical transformation zone. Note the absence of nuclear atypia (H.E. ×100)

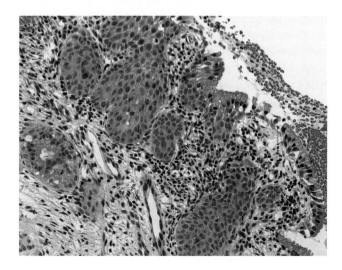

**Fig. 3.6** Transitional cell metaplasia. Note the streaming squamoid cells with nuclear grooves and the absence of high-grade nuclear atypia (H.E. ×200)

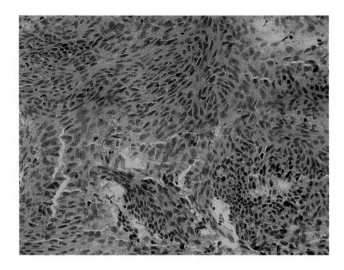

**Fig. 3.7** Naked germinal center. Note the presence of highly active lymphoid cells of germinal center and absence of the mantle zone lymphocytes in this extreme example (H.E. ×200)

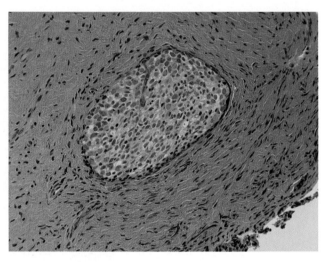

conditions as CIN 2 or 3 will lead to overtreatment of the patient, particularly in the younger age group. Careful examination to exclude significant cytologic atypia/dysplasia is important. Immunohistochemical markers such as P16 and Ki-67 may be helpful in some cases. Typically, a strong cytoplasmic and nuclear staining of P16 along with active mib-1 labeling in both lower and upper epithelium is a feature of high-grade CIN.

## 3.3 Squamous Cell Carcinomas

Microinvasive SCC is defined as early stromal invasion of 5 mm or less in depth. Practically almost always associated with high-grade CIN,

these are small irregular nests of dysplastic epithelial cells that are either highly atypical or individually keratinized. Frequently, nests attached or unattached to the overlying CIN may show abrupt keratinization that is highly suggestive of early invasion (paradoxical maturation). The presence of stromal response is almost always present, including stromal edema, desmoplasia, or prominent inflammatory changes (Fig. 3.8). Another helpful hint for the early stromal invasion is the presence of pseudospaces or clefts between tumor nests and stroma. Findings of definite lymphovascular involvement also confirm an invasive carcinoma. Reporting the actual depth of invasion has been considered to be more useful than a simple diagnosis of microinvasive carcinoma in predicating

**Fig. 3.8** Microinvasive squamous cell carcinoma. Note the abrupt keratinization (paradoxical maturation) and the presence of stromal response (stromal edema, desmoplasia, and prominent inflammatory changes) (H.E. ×40)

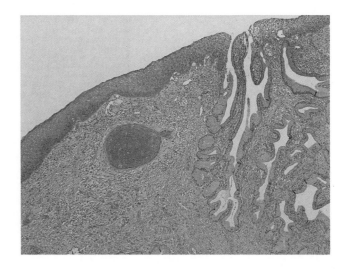

**Fig. 3.9** Squamous cell carcinoma, large cell and keratinizing (H.E. ×40)

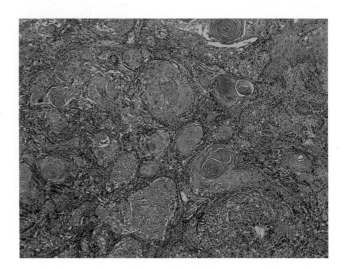

nodal metastasis or long-term prognosis (see AJCC staging).

Conventional SCCs of the cervix include keratinizing, nonkeratinizing, and small cell types. Keratinizing squamous carcinoma consists of sheets and nests of cells having abundant cytoplasm, large nuclei, and inconspicuous nucleoli. Squamous maturation is obvious including keratin pearl formation and the presence of intercellular bridges (Fig. 3.9). Nonkeratinizing type has medium-sized malignant squamous cells with no or minimal keratin production (Fig. 3.10). The small cell carcinoma is a poorly differentiated tumor and consists of confluent sheets of highly atypical, uniformly small round cells with no or minimal desmoplastic stromal response. The tumor cells are cytokeratin positive but evidence of neuroendocrine differentiation is lacking, allowing to distinguish it from the rare small or large cell neuroendocrine carcinomas of the cervix.

In addition, there are well-defined variants of SCC, including basaloid, verrucous, papillary (squamotransitional), lymphoepitheliomatous, and spindle cell or sarcomatoid types. Basaloid carcinoma is an aggressive tumor with characteristic peripheral palisading of the primitive high-grade tumor cells and a lack of stromal response (Fig. 3.11). Verrucous carcinoma is a highly differentiated variant of SCC that is almost indistinguishable from a condyloma or squamous

**Fig. 3.10** Squamous cell carcinoma, large cell and nonkeratinizing (H.E. ×100)

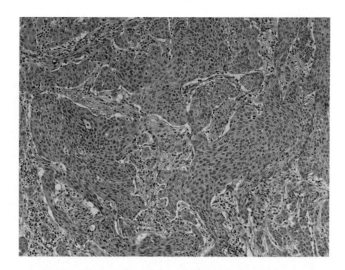

**Fig. 3.11** Basaloid squamous cell carcinoma. Note the peripheral palisading of the primitive high-grade tumor cells within the invasive tumor nests and a lack of stromal response (H.E. ×100)

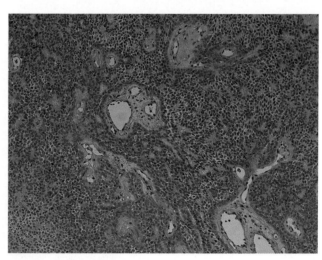

papilloma. Sufficiently large excision may reveal its pushing invasive fronts, eventually leading to the correct diagnosis (see verrucous carcinoma of the vulva). Papillary squamous carcinoma resembles a grade 2 urothelial carcinoma with high-grade dysplastic squamous to focally transitional type cells arranged in papillary growth patterns with stromal cores (Fig. 3.12). The tumor cells express CK7 in almost all cases but 10% also express CK20. The tumor should be sampled extensively for possible coexistence of an underlying invasive component. Lymphoepitheliomatous variant is characterized by syncytial growth of large tumor cells with vesicular nuclei, prominent nucleoli, and surrounding marked inflammatory infiltrates. Spindle cell or sarcomatoid SCC is essentially identical to that of the

upper aerodigestive system. The presence of in situ squamous lesion with focal transition to the spindle component is a helpful hint for correct diagnosis. It should be separated from malignant mixed mullerian tumor, which is often polypoid in gross appearance and contains malignant glandular elements.

## 3.4 Cytology

### 3.4.1 Atypical Squamous Cells

Recognizing our limitations in classifying cytologic changes based on morphology alone, TBS creates the category "atypical squamous cells"

**Fig. 3.12** Papillary squamous cell carcinoma. Note the high-grade dysplastic squamous to focally transitional type cells arranged in a papillary growth patterns with stromal cores (H.E. ×40)

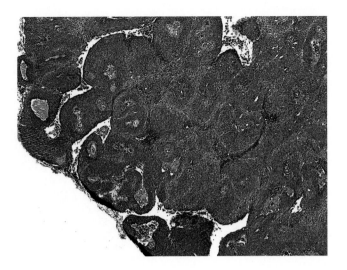

(ASC) to denote "changes suggestive of a squamous intraepithelial lesion that are qualitatively or quantitatively insufficient for a definitive interpretation." The incidence of ASC varies widely from 1.6 to 9.0%. It has been recommended that the frequency of ASC should not be more than 5% or 3× that of SIL. It is important to remember that the category of ASC encompasses a spectrum of cytologic findings and reflects a variety of pathologic process. TBS discourages the use of descriptive terms such as atypical parakeratosis or atypical repair because these terms are not well defined. In addition, TBS 2001 further classifies ASC into two subcategories: atypical squamous cells of undetermined significance (ASC-US) and atypical squamous cells, cannot rule out HSIL (ASC-H).

### 3.4.2 ASC-US

ASC-US is defined as "changes suggestive of a low-grade squamous intraepithelial lesion (LSIL) that are qualitatively or quantitatively insufficient for a definitive interpretation." Despite the definition, about 10–20% of women with ASC-US are found to have a CIN 2 or higher on subsequent follow-up. ASC-US usually involves mature squamous cells. The cytologic criteria for diagnosing ASC-US usually rest on the nuclear features, which include nuclear enlargement – 2.5–3× that of a normal intermediate squamous

cell, mild hyperchromasia, mild chromatin clumping, mild nuclear irregularity, slight increase in N:C ratio, and bi- or multinucleation (Figs. 3.13 and 3.14). Cytoplasmic changes that are associated with HPV infection such as orangeophilic cytoplasm and perinuclear halo are frequently noted. However, these cytoplasmic changes without any accompanying nuclear atypia do not warrant an interpretation of ASC-US. It is important to remember that not all of the criteria need to exist to arrive at an interpretation of ASC-US.

The differential diagnoses include inflammatory and nonneoplastic changes, degenerative changes due to air-drying, and SIL. For specimens showing only nuclear enlargement, a diagnosis of NILM is favored over that of ASC-US if the nuclei appear pale and round with evenly distributed chromatin and smooth nuclear contours. The patient's age, prior history, and HPV status should also be taken into consideration. For women who are peri- or postmenopausal, have had multiple negative Paps previously, or are negative for high-risk HPV, a diagnosis of NILM is favored if the cytologic findings favor a reactive process over a SIL.

### 3.4.3 ASC-H

ASC-H is defined as "changes suggestive of a high-grade squamous intraepithelial lesion

**Fig. 3.13** ASC with nuclear
enlargement and mild
hyperchromasia (ThinPrep.
Papanicolaou, ×400)

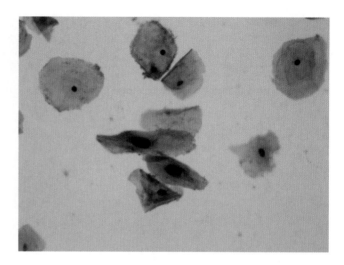

**Fig. 3.14** ASC with
bi/multinucleation.
Intermediate squamous cells
with multinucleation and
nuclear enlargement but
normochromasia and smooth
nuclear membranes
(SurePath, Papanicolaou,
×400)

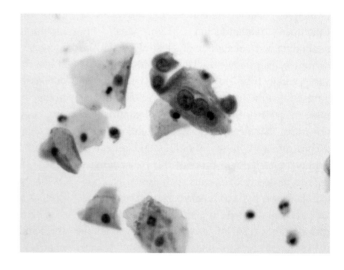

(HSIL) that are qualitatively or quantitatively insufficient for a definitive interpretation." It accounts for less than 10% of all ASC interpretations. ASC-H usually affects immature squamous metaplastic cells. The cells can arrange either singly, in loose cohesive groups, or in cohesive overcrowded clusters. ASC-H cells demonstrate nuclear enlargement – at least 1.5× that of a normal metaplastic cells, high N:C ratio (>50%), coarse chromatin as well as some degree of hyperchromasia, and nuclear membrane irregularity; however, the cellular changes fall short for a definitive diagnosis of HSILs (Fig. 3.15). At other instances, the cells may show bona fide cytologic features of HSIL but there may not be

sufficient number of cells to make a definitive diagnosis of HSIL. Nonneoplastic entities that may be interpreted as ASC-H include histiocytes, degenerated endometrial cells, and atrophic parabasal cells.

One of the variants of ASC-H is "atypical repair." These cells can be immature metaplastic or glandular cells. They differ from the "typical repair" by the presence of considerable nuclear crowding, loosely cohesive group, anisonucleosis, uneven chromatin distribution, irregular nuclear contours, and irregular nucleoli (Fig. 3.16). The differential diagnosis is invasive carcinoma; the lack of conspicuous single atypical cells and tumor diathesis would favor a reactive process.

**Fig. 3.15** ASC, cannot rule out a HSIL. A small group of metaplastic cells showing nuclear enlargement and hyperchromasia. High N:C ratio (>75%) also noted (SurePath, Papanicolaou, ×400)

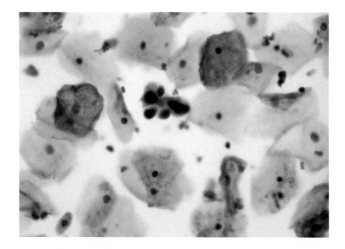

**Fig. 3.16** Atypical repair. Loosely cohesive squamous cells with enlarged nuclei and prominent nucleoli. Considerable degree of anisonucleosis is noted. However, there is no single atypical cells (SurePath, Papanicolaou, ×400)

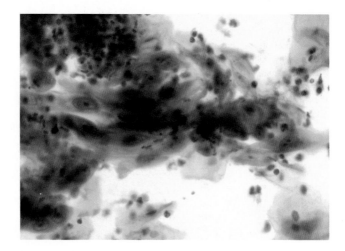

### 3.4.4 Low-Grade Squamous Intraepithelial Lesion

LSIL encompasses lesions that demonstrate HPV cytopathic effects (koilocytosis) and CIN 1 or mild dysplasia. One of the reasons for clumping these two entities together is poor interobserver reproducibility for distinguishing these two cytologically. In addition, the two entities share similar biologic behavior and clinical management.

Both entities usually affect mature squamous cells. The affected cells can occur singly or in sheets. Nuclei are usually enlarged, more than 3× that of intermediate squamous cells, with hyperchromasia, coarse chromatin, and irregular nuclear contours. Nucleoli are infrequently seen. Bi- and multinucleation are common (Fig. 3.17). In addition to the above nuclear changes, koilocytes are

also characterized by the presence of cytoplasmic perinuclear halo, which has a well-defined clear perinuclear zone surrounded by a peripheral rim of densely stained cytoplasm (Fig. 3.18). Parakeratotic (PK) cells with variable degrees of nuclear atypia may be associated with HPV infection, especially if they occur singly or in thick clusters without discernible polarity (Fig. 3.19). On the contrary, PK cells arranging concentrically as squamous pearls or forming aggregates of elongated cells in parallel arrangement are unlikely to be associated with HPV infection.

There is considerable overlap in the cytology between LSIL and ASC-US. In general, LSIL demonstrates more pronounced nuclear atypia than ASC-US. It is also important to distinguish inflammatory halo from koilocytotic halo; the former has ill-defined borders and lacks any

**Fig. 3.17** LSIL. Two intermediate squamous cells with nuclear enlargement (>3×), hyperchromasia, and coarse chromatin. One cell also demonstrates binucleation (SurePath, Papanicolaou, ×400)

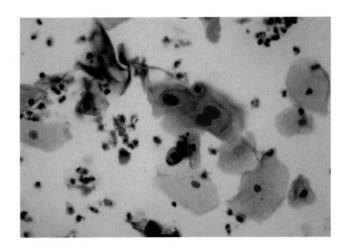

**Fig. 3.18** LSIL (koilocytes). Several intermediate squamous cells with cytoplasmic perinuclear halo and nuclear abnormalities (ThinPrep. Papanicolaou, ×400)

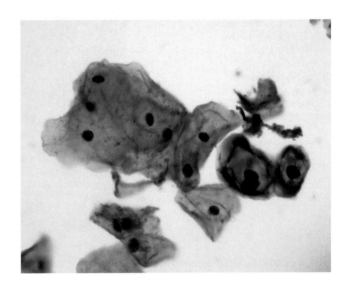

**Fig. 3.19** LSIL with parakeratotic cells in thick cluster with variable degree of nuclear atypia. The cells are arranged in a disordered fashion (SurePath, Papanicolaou, ×400)

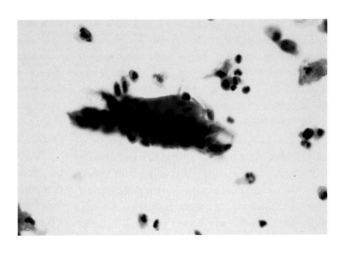

conspicuous nuclear atypia except for nuclear enlargement. Glycogen accumulation in squamous cells can mimic koilocytes; however, nuclear abnormalities are usually absent and the cytoplasm displays a pale yellow tint (Fig. 3.20).

## 3.4.5 High-Grade Squamous Intraepithelial Lesions

According to TBS 2001, HSILs encompass CIN 2 (moderate dysplasia) and CIN 3 (severe dysplasia and carcinoma in situ). HSILs usually present as immature metaplastic or parabasal squamous cells. Individual cells are characterized by marked increased in N:C ratio as a result of nuclear enlargement and a decrease in the cytoplasmic area. The nuclei are enlarged, at least 2× the size of an intermediate squamous cell, and hyperchromatic with coarse chromatin and irregular nuclear membranes (Figs. 3.21 and 3.22). Considerable degree of anisonucleosis is common but nucleoli are infrequent and when present, should raise the suspicious of an invasive carcinoma. Cytoplasm is usually dense and cyanophilic; vacuolation may be noted occasionally. It is quite often that koilocytes and LSIL cells coexist with an HSIL.

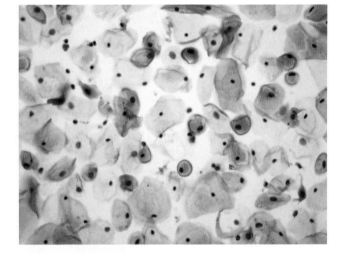

**Fig. 3.20** Glycogen accumulation resulting in cytoplasmic halo, which occupies the entire cells and displays pale yellow tint. No nuclear abnormalities are noted (SurePath, Papanicolaou, ×400)

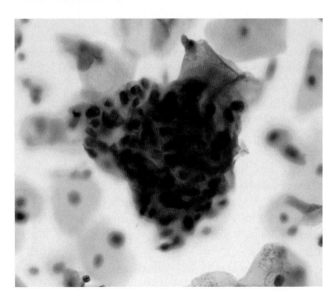

**Fig. 3.21** HSIL. Sheet of metaplastic squamous cells with nuclear enlargement, hyperchromasia, increased N:C ratio, and irregular nuclear contours (SurePath, Papanicolaou, ×400)

**Fig. 3.22** HSIL. Two crowded groups of squamous cells with high N:C ratio and hyperchromatic nuclei (ThinPrep. Papanicolaou, ×400)

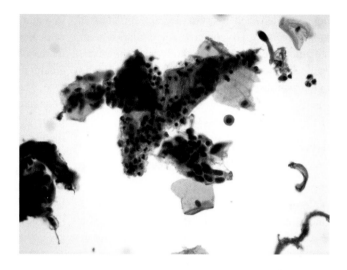

**Fig. 3.23** HSIL. Dysplastic keratinized cells with dense, orangeophilic cytoplasm; increased N:C ratio; hyperchromatic nuclei; and irregular nuclear membrane (SurePath, Papanicolaou, ×400)

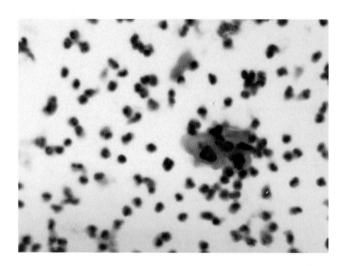

HSIL cells can occur singly, in loosely cohesive groups, crowded sheets, and syncytial aggregates. For conventional preparation, individual HISL cells can also arrange in a single file pattern within mucus strands.

HSIL cells can also present with predominantly keratinized squamous cells with orangeophilic cytoplasm, high N:C ratio, irregular nuclear membranes, and dense and opaque chromatin (Fig. 3.23). Occasionally, these atypical cells can take on a tadpole or spindle shape. Lack of tumor diathesis and nucleoli rule out a keratinizing invasive SCC.

There can be considerable differences in the morphology between LBP and conventional preparation. HSIL cells tend to appear smaller in LBP than those in conventional preparation. In addition, the syncytial aggregates tend to round up and mimic glandular groups in LBP. It is important to note that HSIL cells can appear less hyperchromatic or even normochromatic in LBP.

### 3.4.6 LSIL Cannot Rule Out HSIL

Although TBS only allows two-tier classification for SIL, in some instances, atypical cells may demonstrate features that cannot be classified as LSIL or HSIL. These cells tend to display a slightly higher N:C ratio and/or less mature cytoplasm when compared to typical LSIL cells (Fig. 3.24). In other instances, atypical squamous cells with bona fide features of LSIL are present along with rare cells that are suggestive of HSIL.

### 3.4.7 HSIL with Glandular Involvement

Involvement of the endocervical glands by HSIL is quite common. Cytologically, they present as hyperchromatic crowded groups that are often mistaken as being glandular in origin. Features that favor squamous origin include spindling and whirling of cells in the center of the cluster; flattening of the nuclei at the periphery of the cluster, resulting in a smooth, round border; and coarsely granular chromatin (Fig. 3.25). In addition, the diagnostic features of adenocarcinoma in situ (AIS) are absent and isolated dysplastic squamous cells are often noted in the background. It is important to remember that psuedostratification and nucleoli can be seen in both HSIL involving gland and AIS.

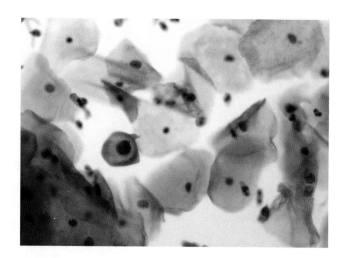

**Fig. 3.24** LSIL cannot rule out HSIL. Atypical squamous cells with increased N:C ratio (>50%) and less mature cytoplasm (SurePath, Papanicolaou, ×400)

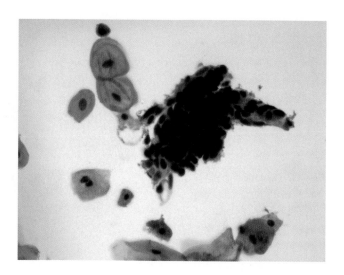

**Fig. 3.25** HSIL with glandular involvement. A crowded group with flattening of the nuclei at one edge resulting in a smooth border. Individual cells demonstrate increased N:C ratio and hyperchromatic nuclei (SurePath, Papanicolaou, ×400)

### 3.4.8 Squamous Cell Carcinoma

Although TBS does not require subclassifying of SCC, it is helpful to discuss the cytologic features of various subtypes of SCC separately. Keratinizing SCC is characterized by keratinized squamous cells with bizarre shapes such as tadpole, caudate, and spindle shape. Nuclei are enlarged, pleomorphic, and hyperchromatic; nucleoli are usually not apparent (Figs. 3.26 and 3.27). N:C ratio is increased but much lower than that of HSIL. The atypical squamous cells are often seen isolated and, less frequently, in small aggregates.

Nonkeratinizing SCC is characterized by crowded aggregates of large round to oval cells with moderate amount of cyanophilic cytoplasm and increased N:C ratio. Syncytial arrangement is common. In contrast to the previous subtype, nucleoli are usually large and prominent. Chromatin is coarsely granular and unevenly distributed. Single cells are not infrequent (Figs. 3.28 and 3.29).

SCC, small cell variant, is characterized by cohesive aggregates of small cells with scant nondescript cytoplasm and very high N:C ratio. Nuclear molding is frequent. Nucleoli are inconspicuous. According to TBS, this subtype of SCC is classified under the category of "other malignancies." The differential diagnosis includes follicular cervicitis, which demonstrates mostly isolated cells with a mixture of small and large lymphocytes and tingible body macrophages.

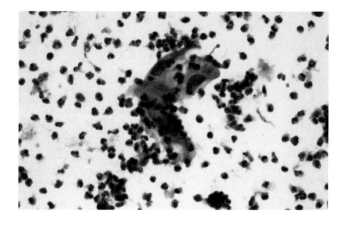

**Fig. 3.26** Keratinizing SCC. Bizarre keratinized squamous with pleomorphic, hyperchromatic nuclei and moderate amount of orangeophilic cytoplasm (SurePath, Papanicolaou, ×400)

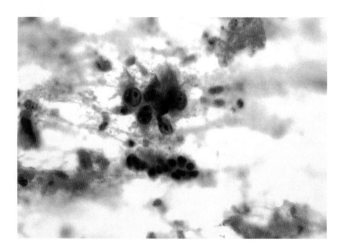

**Fig. 3.27** Keratinizing SCC. A small group of dyskaryotic squamous cells with prominent nucleoli in a hemorrhagic background (conventional preparation, Papanicolaou, ×400)

**Fig. 3.28** Nonkeratinizing SCC. Syncytial aggregate of squamous cells with marked increased in N:C ratio and hyperchromatic nuclei. Distinct nucleoli are noted in scattered cells. The cytoplasm is scant and cyanophilic with indistinct cell borders (SurePath, Papanicolaou, ×400)

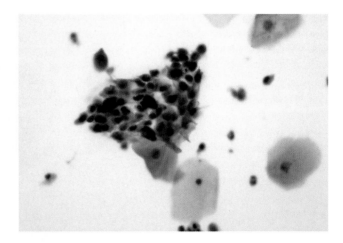

**Fig. 3.29** Nonkeratinizing SCC. Dyscohesive malignant squamous cells admixed with amorphous debris and inflammatory cells (conventional preparation, Papanicolaou, ×400)

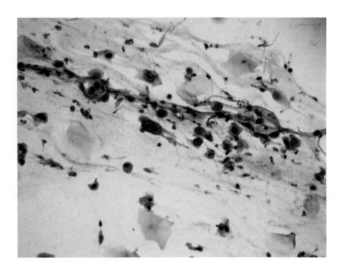

One feature that is common to all three subtypes of SCC is the presence of tumor diathesis, which is composed on necrotic debris, old blood, and inflammation (Fig. 3.30). However, not all SCCs demonstrate tumor diathesis. In addition, malignant cells may be scarce and obscured by debris and inflammation. For LBP, tumor diathesis tends to be present at the periphery of the cellular clusters, instead of distributing throughout the slides.

In the absence of convincing tumor diathesis and/or conspicuous nucleoli, it may be difficult to distinguish SCC from HSIL. When dealing with such a situation, TBS recommends using the diagnostic term "HSIL with features suggestive of invasive carcinoma."

### 3.4.9  Mimics of Neoplastic Diseases

According to the TBS 2001, any benign and nonneoplastic findings are classified under the category of "Negative of intraepithelial lesion and malignancy." In addition, the current TBS prefers the category of "organisms" to "infections" because the presence of some organisms may reflect colonization rather than clinical infection. Furthermore, except for the microorganisms listed in TBS, the reporting of other benign and nonneoplastic findings is optional. However, it is still important to recognize these changes because many changes can mimic preneoplastic and malignant lesions.

**Fig. 3.30** Tumor diathesis
consisting of necrotic debris
and inflammatory cells tend
to be clumped in liquid-based
preparation. A nearby cluster
of neoplastic squamous cells
(ThinPrep. Papanicolaou,
×200)

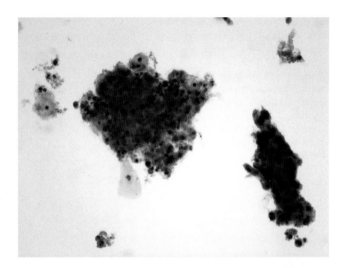

**Fig. 3.31** Lactobacilli with
cytolysis. Numerous bacterial
rods are noted in the
background. There are also
several naked nuclei devoid
of cytoplasm (SurePath,
Papanicolaou, ×400)

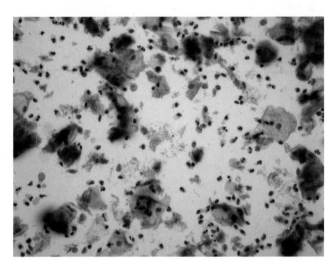

### 3.4.9.1 Microorganisms

Infectious vaginitis is one of the most common women's healthcare problems worldwide. The three leading agents that are responsible for 90% of infectious vaginitis are bacterial vaginosis (BV) and candidiasis, and Trichomonas vaginalis. Other microorganisms that may cause infectious vaginitis include herpes simplex virus (HSV), actinomyces, chylamydia, and gonorrhea.

### 3.4.9.2 Bacterial Organisms

Lactobacilli spp. occurs in 20% of screened women, especially in abundance during luteal phase and pregnancy, as well as in women receiving exogenous hormonal treatment (Fig. 3.31). They appear as rod of variable length. They may cause lysis of glycogen-rich intermediate squamous cells, resulting in numerous bare nuclei.

BV is characterized by a mixed infection of anaerobic bacteria; *Gardnerella vaginalis* is considered to be one of the major bacteria causing this infection. In conventional preparation, the background is diffusely covered by small cocci, whereas in LBP, the background is usually clean with scattered clusters of cocci. In both preparations, the bacteria adhere diffusely and evenly to the surface of the squamous cells, which are referred to as clue cells (Fig. 3.32). There is also a conspicuous absence of lactobacilli. The recommended TBS interpretation is "shift in flora suggestive of bacterial vaginosis."

Actinomyces species are often associated with women wearing an intrauterine contraceptive device (IUD); up to 25% of women with IUD will have actinomyces present in their Pap specimens. They appear densely clustered with thin filamentous organisms radiating from the edges of the clusters, resembling a cotton ball (Fig. 3.33). The background can be clean or inflammatory.

The cellular changes associated with infection with *Chlamydia trachomatis* include the presence of cytoplasmic vacuoles that often group around the nucleus. Small eosinophilic bodies may be found within the vacuoles (Fig. 3.34). Unfortunately, these changes are nonspecific. As a result, TBS does not recommend diagnosing *C. trachomatis* infection based on morphology alone.

### 3.4.9.3  Fungal Organisms

Most cases of fungal vaginal infection are caused by Candida species. The organisms appear as budding yeast and pseudohyphae, often in a background of acute inflammation. Squamous cells can display ill-defined cytoplasmic clearing,

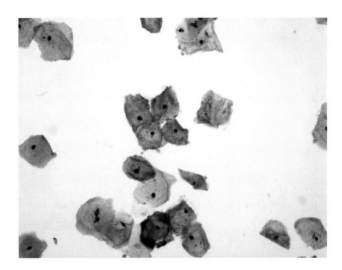

**Fig. 3.32** Clue cells. Superficial squamous cells are covered diffusely by bacterial cocci. Note that the background is usually clean in liquid-based preparation (ThinPrep. Papanicolaou, ×400)

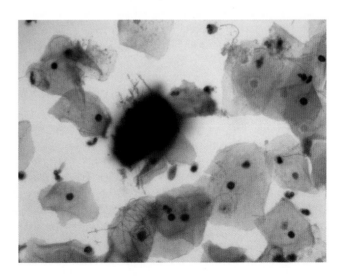

**Fig. 3.33** Actinomyces. Colony of filamentous bacteria, resembling a cotton ball (SurePath, Papanicolaou, ×400)

**Fig. 3.34** Changes
suggestive of Chlamydial
infection. One of the
endocervical/metaplastic cells
displays a large cytoplasmic
vacuole with inclusions
(ThinPrep. Papanicolaou,
×400)

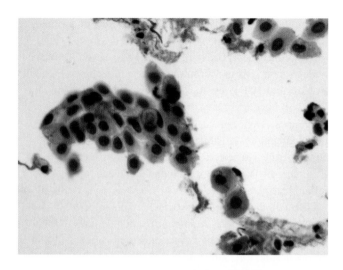

**Fig. 3.35** Candida.
Pseudohyphae are noted in an
inflammatory background.
A row of squamous cells
appeared to be "speared" by
fungal pseudohyphae
(SurePath, Papanicolaou,
×400)

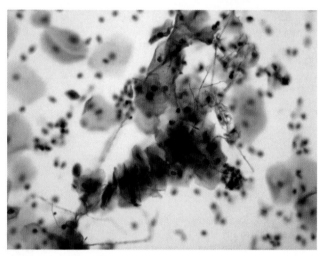

resulting in a moth-eaten appearance. Another characteristic feature is that a row of squamous cells appears to be "speared" by fungal pseudohyphae, resembling a "shish kebab" (Fig. 3.35).

### 3.4.9.4 Viral Organisms

The most common viral infection of the female genital tract is caused by HPV, which has been discussed earlier in the chapter. HSVs, both I and II, can also infect the female genital tract. Squamous cells infected by HSV are characterized by 3Ms – multinucleation, margination of the chromatin (resulting in a ground glass appearance), and molding of the nuclei (Fig. 3.36). Another characteristic of HSV infection is the presence of a large intranuclear inclusion surrounded by a halo. The background is usually inflammatory and necrotic. Reactive and reparative changes in the squamous cells are frequently observed.

### 3.4.9.5 Parasitic Organisms

*Trichomonas vaginalis* accounts for the majority of the sexually transmitted parasitic infections. The organisms appear as bluish-gray, ovoid to pear-shaped structures, measuring 15–30 μm in size. Identifying the presence of a small, dense eccentric nucleus and/or small red cytoplasmic granules avoids mistaking detached cytoplasmic

**Fig. 3.36** Herpes simplex virus. Multiple nucleated giant cells with the characteristic ground-glass chromatin. Nuclear molding and margination of the chromatin are noted. There are also intranuclear inclusions (SurePath, Papanicolaou, ×400)

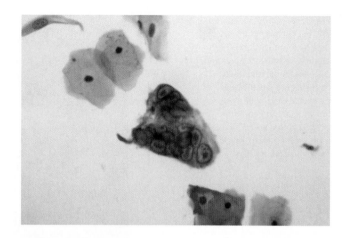

**Fig. 3.37** Trichomonas. Pear-shaped, bluish-gray organism with small red cytoplasmic granules (*circle*). An example of "poly ball," squamous cell covered by numerous neutrophils is noted in the *upper right-hand corner* and an example of squamous cells with a vague small perinuclear halo in the *upper left-hand corner* (SurePath, Papanicolaou, ×400)

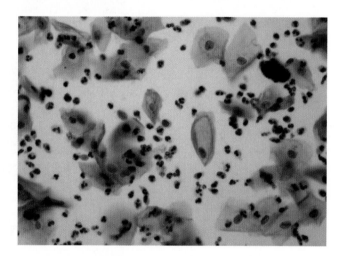

fragments as trichomonads (Fig. 3.37). Leptothrix, a thin, elongated bacterium, may accompany trichomonads. Accompanying squamous cells often demonstrate small perinuclear halos or are surrounded by numerous neutrophils, known as "poly balls."

### 3.4.9.6 Noninfectious Cervicovaginitis

#### 3.4.9.6.1 Atrophic Vaginitis

Atrophic vaginitis usually occurs in postmenopausal women and rarely in postpartum women. For conventional preparation, the background is usually characterized by inflammation and granular debris simulating tumor diathesis (Fig. 3.38). For LBP, inflammatory cells and granular debris

tend to clump together, resulting in a relatively clean background. The predominant cell type is parabasal cell, which can arrange either singly or in large monolayer sheets with preserved nuclear polarity (Fig. 3.39). Individual cells can display nuclear enlargement, up to 3× that of an intermediate squamous cell, mild hyperchromasia, and more elongated nuclei. Other features include blue blobs (basophilic globular amorphous materials) and pseudo-PK cells (degenerated parabasal cells with pyknotic nuclei and orangeophilic cytoplasm).

#### 3.4.9.6.2 Keratinization

The squamous epithelium of the cervix and upper two-thirds of the vagina is nonkeratinized.

**Fig. 3.38** Atrophic vaginitis. The background is characterized by granular debris with scattered parabasal squamous cells. Psuedoparakeratotic cells that are degenerated parabasal cells with pyknotic nuclei and orangeophilic cytoplasm are noted (conventional preparation, Papanicolaou, ×400)

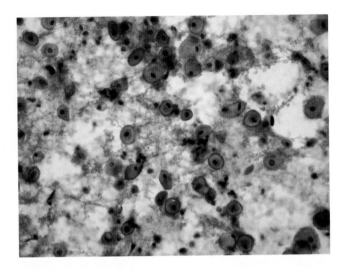

**Fig. 3.39** Atrophy. Large fragments of parabasal cells presented as hyperchromatic crowded group. Preservation of nuclear polarity helps in the differential diagnosis (SurePath, Papanicolaou, ×400)

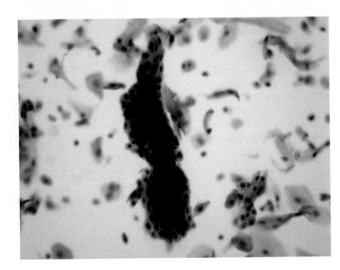

Keratinization can occur as a response to a chronic irritation of benign nature such as inflection or uterine prolapse; rarely, keratinization can be associated with a dysplastic or malignant process. One manifestation is hyperkeratosis, which is represented by the presence of anucleated squamous cells (ANSC), i.e., mature polygonal squamous cells that are devoid of nuclei; empty spaces or "ghost nuclei" may be seen (Fig. 3.40). Another manifestation is parakeratosis, which is characterized by the presence of small superficial squamous cells with intense orangeophilic cytoplasm. The PK squamous cells can occur singly, in small clusters, in large sheets, or as squamous pearls. Nuclei are usually small and pyknotic

(Figs. 3.41 and 3.42). The presence of either ANSC or PK does not warrant reporting but should alert the cytologist to look carefully for the possibility of a more serious lesion. Furthermore, the finding of PK cells with nuclear atypia should be diagnosed as epithelial cell abnormality and necessitate a careful search for koilocytes and/or dysplastic squamous cells (Fig. 3.43).

### 3.4.9.6.3 Reactive Cellular Changes (Including Repair)

Reactive cellular changes can be associated with inflammation, infection, therapeutic effects,

**Fig. 3.40** Hyperkeratosis. Clusters of anucleated squames devoid of any nuclei (ThinPrep, Papanicolaou, ×400)

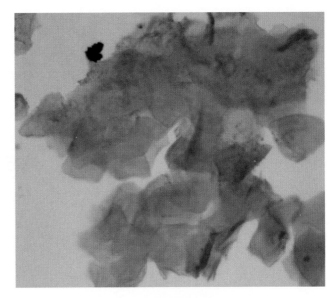

**Fig. 3.41** Parakeratosis. Strips of small superficial squamous cells with intense opaque orangeophilic cytoplasm (SurePath, Papanicolaou, ×400)

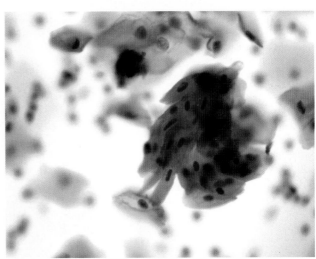

**Fig. 3.42** Parakeratosis. Parakeratotic squamous cells arranged in a concentric circle, resulting in a squamous pearl (SurePath, Papanicolaou, ×400)

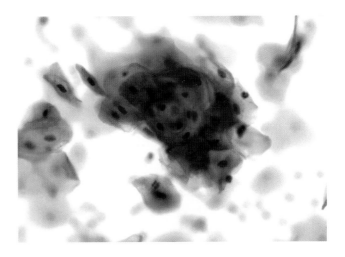

**Fig. 3.43** Atypical parakeratotis. Parakeratotic squamous cells with nuclear enlargement and irregular nuclear contours. This should be classified as ASC under the current TBS (SurePath, Papanicolaou, ×400)

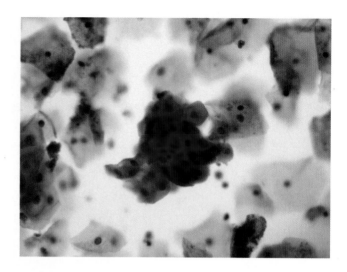

**Fig. 3.44** Reactive cellular changes. Metaplastic squamous cells showing mild nuclear enlargement and small perinuclear cytoplasmic halos with poorly defined borders. A reactive intermediate squamous cell demonstrating binucleation (SurePath, Papanicolaou, ×400)

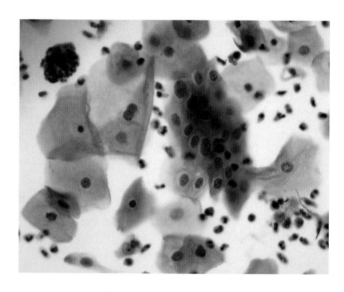

mechanical irritation, neoplasia, or other nonspecific etiologies. Reactive squamous cells, affecting both intermediate and metaplastic cells, usually demonstrate nuclear enlargement up to 2× that of an intermediate squamous cell (Fig. 3.44). Mild hyperchromasia may be evident but the chromatin remains finely granular and evenly distributed. Nuclear outlines are smooth and round. Distinct nucleoli may be present, particularly with LBP. Binucleation is not infrequent. Cytoplasm may show polychromasia, vacuolization,

or perinuclear halos without peripheral thickening. The N:C ratio remains normal.

Reparative changes are characterized by flat, monolayer sheets of cells that are often streaming in one direction. There is usually abundant cytoplasm that is often drawn out, resembling cell culture (Fig. 3.45). These features are more pronounced in conventional preparation, whereas the cells are more rounded with less streaming in LBP. The nuclei are often enlarged, resulting in slightly increased N:C ratio. The nuclear membranes are

**Fig. 3.45** Repair. Flat, monolayer, cohesive sheet of squamous cells with normal N:C ratio, nuclear enlargement, vesicular chromatin, and prominent nucleoli (SurePath, Papanicolaou, ×400)

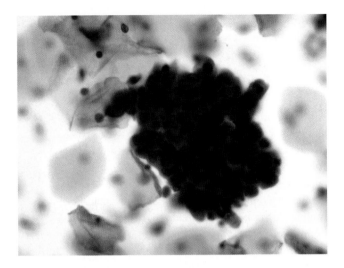

**Fig. 3.46** Therapeutic changes. Very large and bizarre squamous cells with nuclear enlargement. However, the N:C ratio remains low and the nuclear chromatin appears smudged (conventional preparation, Papanicolaou, ×400)

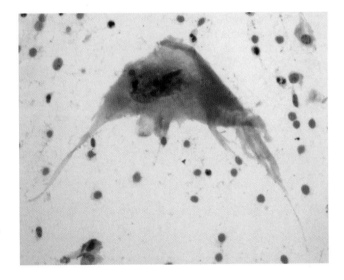

uniform and the nucleoli are round, prominent, and, sometimes, multiple. Infiltration of the sheets by neutrophils is frequently noted. Occasional mitotic figures may be seen. Single cells with nuclear atypia are typically absent. The differential diagnosis includes invasive carcinoma.

### 3.4.9.6.4   Therapeutic Changes

Cellular changes induced by radiation and chemotherapy include cytomegaly without an increase in N:C ratio, nuclear enlargement, bi- or multinucleation, cytoplasmic vacuolization with or without inflammatory cells, and cytoplasmic polychromasia (Fig. 3.46). The chromatin often appears dark and smudged. Multinucleated histiocytes and a mixture of inflammatory cells can be seen in the background. Therapy-induced changes can last for years after the initial treatment; therefore, it is important to provide any past history of radiation and chemotherapy. Similar changes can also been seen in patients with folate and vitamin B12 deficiency. It can be quite difficult to distinguish between therapeutic effects and carcinoma; increase in N:C ratio, irregularly distributed, coarsely granular chromatin, and keratinization, when present, favor the latter.

### 3.4.9.6.5 Artifacts

Air-drying artifacts due to delay in fixation are usually limited to conventional preparation. Air-dried cells tend to be larger than their well-preserved counterpart with pale cytoplasm and smudged nuclei, resulting in a washed-out appearance. The finding of normal N:C ratio and smooth nuclear contours favors benign air-dried cells over dysplastic air-dried cells.

Cornflaking is due to drying of the mounting media prior to coverslipping, resulting in air bubbles trapped between the coverslip and the cells. Microscopically, the air bubbles appear as coarse, dark brown refractile granules.

## 3.5 Clinical Staging and Management

AJCC Cancer Staging Manual (Seventh Edition, 2010) Staging of cervical cancers (including both squamous and glandular lesions).

## Suggested Reading

Clement PB, Young RH. Atlas of Gynecologic Surgical Pathology. 2nd Edition. Saunders, Philadelphia, PA. 2008.

Diane S, Nayar R, Davey DD, and Wilbur DC. The Bethesda System for Reporting Cervical Cytology: Definitions, Criteria, and Explanatory Notes. 2nd Edition. Springer, Berlin. 2004.

Kurman R. Blaustein's Pathology of the Female Genital Tract. 5th Edition. Springer, Berlin. 2002.

# Chapter 4
# Glandular Lesions of the Cervix

**Keywords** Cervix • Polyp • Glandular abnormalities • Adenocarcinoma in situ • Invasive adenocarcinoma

## 4.1 Cervical Polyp and Other Tumor-Like Conditions

*Endocervical polyp* is usually single and less than 1 cm in size. Histologically, the polyp consists of varying proportions of squamous and endocervical epithelium, and stromal components. The overall appearance can be adenomatous, cystic, fibrous, or inflammatory. Surface ulceration or involvement by CIN or adenocarcinoma may be seen.

*Tunnel cluster* is a localized proliferation of endocervical glands, commonly seen in multigravid women. Type A tunnel cluster is well circumscribed and noncystic. It consists of crowded endocervical glands in lobules. Irregular glands with mild atypia may be seen, but mitotic activity is generally absent. Type B lesion is expansile or lobular, with dilated glands that are covered by more flattened cells (Fig. 4.1). The lesion may involve deeper cervical stroma. The absence of significant cytologic atypia, mitosis, and deep infiltrative growth separates tunnel clusters from adenocarcinomas.

*Deep Nabothian cysts* manifest as deep-seated, cystically dilated, mucin-filled endocervical glands. Extravasated mucin pool may be present. The lack of a mass lesion, infiltrative glands, and

unequivocal malignant cells separates it from the minimal deviation adenocarcinoma.

*Lobular and diffuse glandular hyperplasias* are benign mucinous glandular proliferations, either lobular or diffuse. They may be more than 1.0 cm, deep-seated into the cervical stroma. Both show crowded endocervical glands with lining mucin-producing cells (Fig. 4.2). Cytologic atypia is mild in general, but mitotic activity (2/10 HPF) can be found in some cases. In diffuse hyperplasia, although confluent in growth pattern, the demarcation from the stroma is sharp and smooth. The superficial location, noninfiltrative border, the absence of definite malignant cells, and desmoplastic stromal response are important features in their separation from a minimal deviation adenocarcinoma. In very rare cases, the hyperplasia may have borderline features with less well-defined border and certain cytologic atypia. Some authors believe that these may represent precursor lesions of minimal deviation adenocarcinoma.

*Microglandular hyperplasia* (MGH) is traditionally considered as a hormonally related lesion of the cervix in patients receiving progesterone. Most are incidental polypoid lesions consisting of closely packed small- to medium-sized endocervical glands with inconspicuously intervening stroma. Uniform endocervical cells with subnuclear vacuoles, associated squamous metaplasia, focal reserve cell proliferation imparting double-layered epithelium, and the presence of many neutrophils in the stroma are characteristic. Mild nuclear atypia

D. Chhieng and P. Hui (eds.), *Cytology and Surgical Pathology of Gynecologic Neoplasms,*
Current Clinical Pathology, DOI 10.1007/978-1-60761-164-6_4,
© Springer Science+Business Media, LLC 2011

**Fig. 4.1** Tunnel cluster. Note the expansile or larger lobules with dilated glands that are covered by more flattened cells (H.E. ×40)

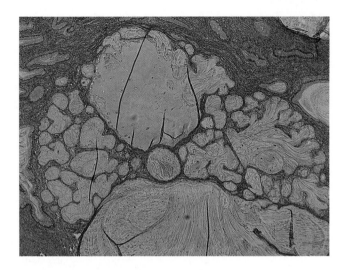

**Fig. 4.2** Lobular endocervical glandular hyperplasia. Note the lobulated, crowded endocervical glands with lining mucin-producing cells (H.E. ×40)

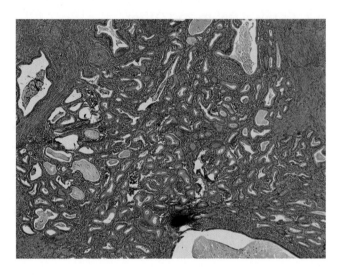

may be present, so are occasional mitotic figures (Fig. 4.3a, b). The absence of infiltrative growth and no more than mild cytologic atypia separate it from adenocarcinoma, particularly the clear cell carcinoma. Separation from an endometrial microglandular adenocarcinoma can be difficult, particularly if the lesional tissue is not associated with background endometrium. Fractional curettage may be helpful, but not so as by immunohistochemistry.

*Chronic endocervicitis* may present with intense lymphoid hyperplasia with marked squamous metaplasia and secondary lymphoid follicle formation. Surface papillary epithelial proliferation with associated lymphoid follicles is sometimes called "papillary cervicitis." Not infrequently, the lymphoid germinal center may be confused with high-grade squamous intraepithelial lesions (see Chap. 3, Fig. 3.7).

*Arias-Stella reaction* may involve endocervical mucosa or an endocervical polyp. It tends to be focal and strikingly papillary. The reactive cells may be enlarged and have abundant clear cytoplasm and epically located hyperchromatic nuclei (hobnail cells) closely resembling those of a clear cell carcinoma. The degenerative nature

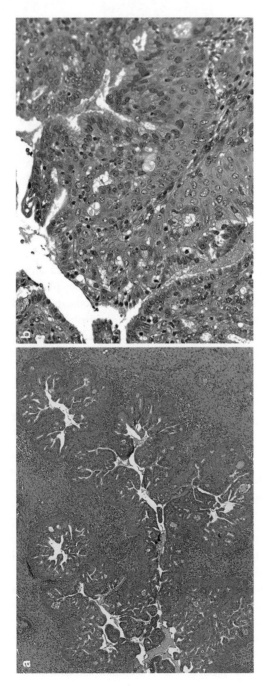

**Fig. 4.3** Microglandular hyperplasia. The lesions consist of closely packed small- to medium-sized endocervical glands with inconspicuously intervening stroma (**a**, H.E. ×40). Uniform endocervical cells with subnuclear vacuoles, associated squamous metaplasia, focal reserve cell proliferation imparting double-layered epithelium, and the presence of many neutrophils (**b**, H.E. ×200)

**Fig. 4.4** Arias-Stella reaction. Note the enlarged glandular epithelial cells with abundant clear cytoplasm and epically located hyperchromatic nuclei (hobnail cells) (H.E. ×200)

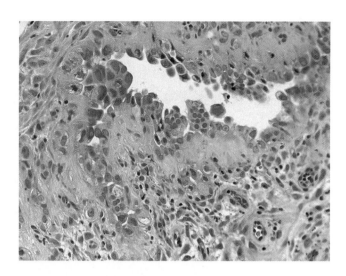

of the nuclei and absence of mitosis and knowledge of pregnancy or hormonal use are features of Arias-Stella reaction (Fig. 4.4).

*Endometriosis, endosalpingiosis, and tubal metaplasia* are frequently encountered benign alterations of the cervix. Mesonephric hyperplasia is typically found at the lateral sides of the cervix and consists of proliferation in a lobular or irregular distribution around a centrally located duct (Fig. 4.5a). The cuboidal epithelial cells and the presence of luminal eosinophilic secretion are characteristic (Fig. 4.5b).

## 4.2  Glandular Dysplasia/ Adenocarcinoma In Situ

Three morphologic types of in situ adenocarcinoma have been described, including endocervical (>80%, Fig. 4.6), intestinal (Fig. 4.7), and endometrioid (Fig. 4.8) adenocarcinomas. All the three histologic types have the following morphologic features: (1) cellular crowding with nuclear stratification, (2) moderate to serve nuclear atypia including hyperchromatia and nuclear megaly, and (3) readily identifiable mitotic figures and apoptotic bodies. Additional features include epithelial branching, budding, or cribriforming. Lesions with one or two of the above three criteria may be interpreted as glandular

dysplasia, although some authors recommend not reporting such due to a lack of understanding of their biology and clinical behavior. Squamous intraepithelial neoplasia commonly coexists with adenocarcinoma in situ (AIS) (80%). Rare forms of intraepithelial tumors include ciliated, adenosquamous, and even serous and clear cell in situ lesions.

## 4.3  Invasive Adenocarcinomas

Invasive adenocarcinoma of the cervix now represents 10–20% of all cervical cancers. Similar to squamous carcinoma, it affects primarily patients aged 50 years or above, and high-risks HPVs, particularly type 18, are causal agents for most of the cases. Mesonephric adenocarcinoma and mucinous minimal deviation adenocarcinoma appear unrelated to HPV infection. Minimal deviation mucinous adenocarcinoma is associated with Peutz–Jeghers syndrome in some patients.

*Usual endocervical adenocarcinoma* represents 80–90% of all cervical adenocarcinomas. The tumor is characterized by a proliferation of medium-size glands with tumor cells that have eosinophilic to amphophilic cytoplasm with no or minimal mucin production (Fig. 4.9a). Angulated to cribriforming glands with high nuclear

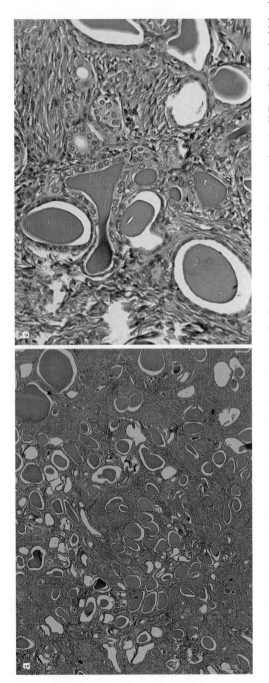

**Fig. 4.5** Mesonephric hyperplasia. Note the glandular proliferation in lobular or irregular distribution around a centrally located duct (**a**, H.E. ×40), the cuboidal epithelial cells and the presence of luminal eosinophilic secretion (**b**, H.E. ×200)

**Fig. 4.6** Endocervical
adenocarcinoma in situ,
conventional type (H.E. ×200)

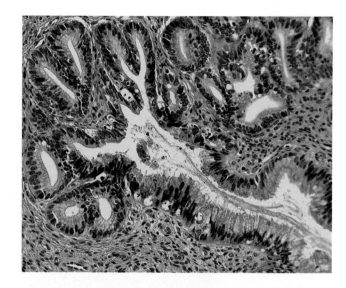

**Fig. 4.7** Endocervical
adenocarcinoma in situ,
intestinal type. Note the
presence of goblet cells
(H.E. ×200)

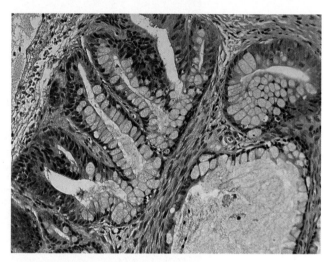

**Fig. 4.8** Endocervical
adenocarcinoma in situ,
endometrioid type
(H.E. ×200)

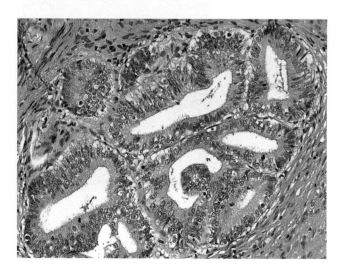

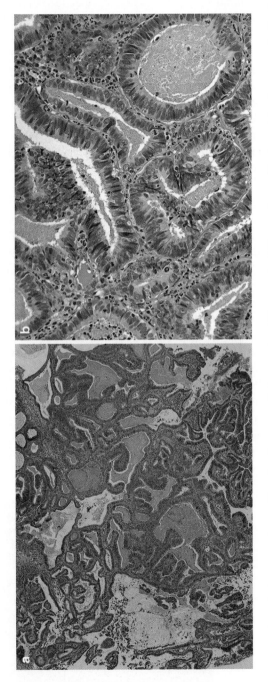

**Fig. 4.9** Usual type endocervical adenocarcinoma. Note that the tumor cells have eosinophilic to amphophilic cytoplasm with no or minimal mucin production (**a**, H.E. ×40), and angulated to cribriforming glands with high nuclear grade, brisk mitotic activity, and conspicuous apoptotic bodies (**b**, H.E. ×200)

grade, brisk mitotic activity and conspicuous apoptotic bodies are characteristic (Fig. 4.9b). Variations of the glandular architecture are common, including cribriforming, infiltrative, cystic, microglandular, papillary, and solid growth patterns. Unlike squamous lesions, there is a lack of uniform agreement regarding the diagnostic criteria and the clinical management for microinvasive adenocarcinoma of the cervix. Diagnosis of some early invasive adenocarcinoma relies on pattern recognition, i.e., abnormal glands showing growth configurations incompatible with the normal glandular distribution (Fig. 4.10). Continuous or band-like growth of dysplastic glands involving large areas of cervical mucosa is a feature of invasive adenocarcinoma. Inter- and intraglandular complexities, including closely packed glands, marked variations of gland size and shape, and extensive cribriforming, are highly suspicious for invasion. Deeply seated glands or glands with close approximation to larger vasculature also suggest invasion (Fig. 4.11). In some early invasive lesions, budding of single or clusters of dysplastic cells from an in situ adenocarcinoma along with stromal response is diagnostic of early invasion (Fig. 4.12).

*Villoglandular adenocarcinoma* commonly occurs in young women with average age 40 years. The tumor presents as a polypoid friable mass. Histologically, it is characterized by long and slender papillae, covered with mild to moderately atypical cells of endocervical origin or endometrioid type in rare cases. The epithelium is flat without tufting (Fig. 4.13). Most are exophytic tumors without deep stromal invasion. However, a biopsy diagnosis of villoglandular adenocarcinoma should be followed by hysterectomy to rule out underlying invasive adenocarcinoma. Conservative treatment may be reserved for those who have had a cone excision that contains the entire lesion without underlying stromal invasion, lymphovascular and margin involvement.

*Endometrioid adenocarcinoma* is rare and may be associated with cervical endometriosis. Its differential diagnosis with an endometrial primary carcinoma largely depends on the location of the tumor. Clinical findings, fraction curettage, immunohistochemistry (P16, CEA vimentin, and ER), and HPV testing are helpful in most cases. An endocervical primary adenocarcinoma has tumor cells typically positive for HPV, CEA and P16, but negative for vimentin and ER. An endometrial primary adenocarcinoma typically shows the opposite immunohistochemical profile: positive for vimentin and ER, but negative for HPV, CEA and P16.

*Minimal deviation adenocarcinoma (adenoma maligna)* is a rare mucinous carcinoma that it is frequently overlooked due to its deceptively benign-looking glands (Fig. 4.14a, b). There is a generally haphazard distribution of open glands of highly variable sizes and shapes.

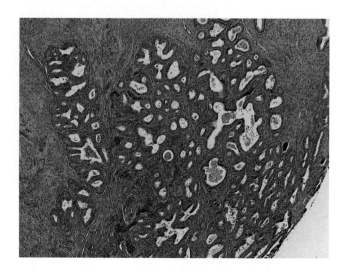

**Fig. 4.10** Early invasive adenocarcinoma. Note the continuous or band-like growth patterns of dysplastic glands involving large areas of cervical mucosa (H.E. ×40)

**Fig. 4.11** Early invasive adenocarcinoma. Note the deeply seated glands or glands with close approximation to larger vasculature (H.E. ×200)

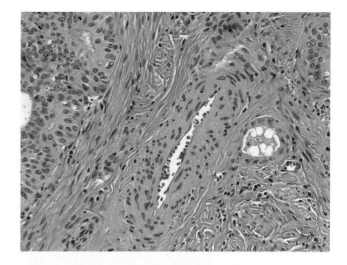

**Fig. 4.12** Early invasive adenocarcinoma. Note the budding of single or clusters of dysplastic cells from the in situ adenocarcinoma along with a stromal response (H.E. ×20)

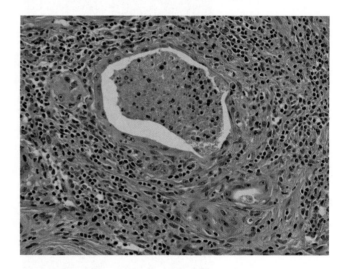

**Fig. 4.13** Villoglandular adenocarcinoma of the cervix (H.E. ×100)

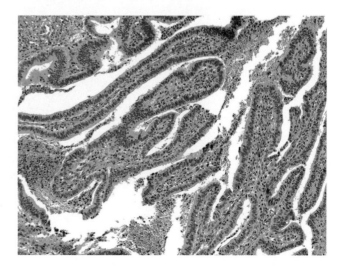

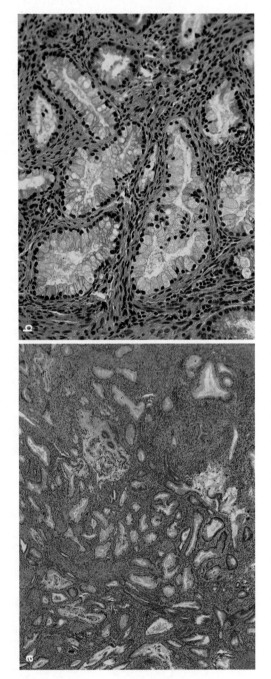

**Fig. 4.14** (**a**, **b**) Minimal deviation adenocarcinoma. Note the deceptively benign-looking mucinous glands that are haphazardly distributed (**a**, H.E. ×40, **b**, H.E. ×200)

The lesion may be deeply invasive, which may not be appreciated in a small biopsy. High index of suspicion is important and careful histologic examination usually reveals definite dysplastic glands and/or single or clusters of infiltrating tumor cells with stromal response. Other helpful hints include close juxtaposition of glands to larger vasculatures and the presence of lymphovascular and perineural invasion.

*Endocervical and intestinal-type mucinous adenocarcinomas* are recognized by their obvious intracellular mucin production. True endocervical adenocarcinoma of the mucinous type is well differentiated with overall architectural and cytologic features of the usual type, with additional presence of abundant intracytoplasmic mucin (Fig. 4.15). Some authors believe that most minimal deviation adenocarcinomas fit to this category as well. The intestinal-type mucinous adenocarcinomas resemble those of large intestine and are histologically characterized by the presence of goblet cells and occasionally argentaffin and Paneth cells (Fig. 4.16). Rare cervical primary signet-ring cell adenocarcinoma has been reported.

*Glassy cell carcinoma* is considered as a poorly differentiated variant of adenocarcinoma or adenosquamous carcinoma. Over 80% of the

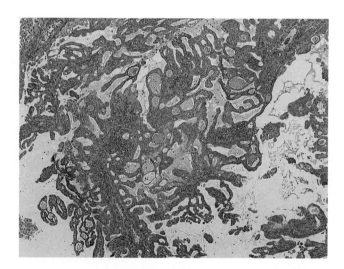

**Fig. 4.15** Mucinous microglandular adenocarcinoma of the cervix (H.E. ×40)

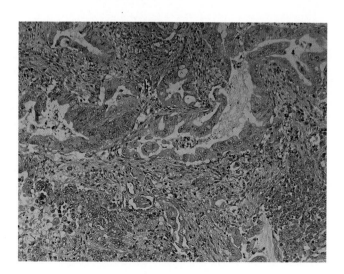

**Fig. 4.16** Mucinous intestinal adenocarcinoma of the cervix. Note the presence of goblet cells (H.E. ×100)

**Fig. 4.17** Glassy cell
carcinoma. Note the sheets
of large, poorly differentiated
cells that are rich in
eosinophilic or amphophilic
cytoplasm, imparting a
ground-glass appearance
(H.E. ×200)

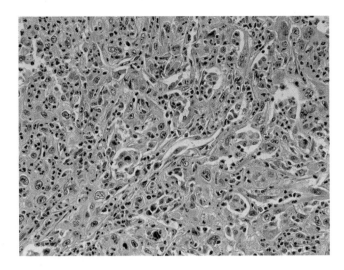

**Fig. 4.18** Adenosquamous
carcinoma. Note the
well-developed glandular
structures within the
squamous tumor nests
(H.E. ×200)

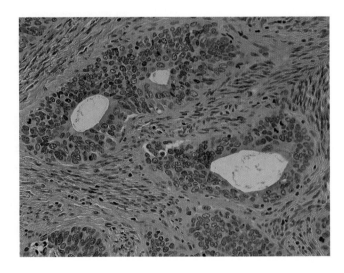

cases are seen in patients younger than 35 years of age. The tumor is characterized by sheets of large, poorly differentiated cells that are rich in eosinophilic or amphophilic cytoplasm, imparting a ground-glass appearance. Distinct cell membrane, large round nuclei with prominent macronucleoli, and the presence of dense inflammatory infiltrates (eosinophils and lymphoplasma cells) are typical findings (Fig. 4.17).

*Adenosquamous carcinoma* is defined by the presence of malignant tumor nests with both squamous and glandular differentiation. Unequivocal glandular differentiation must be seen for the diagnosis (Fig. 4.18). Focal squamous

differentiation (metaplasia) in a typical adenocarcinoma, the presence of clear cell carcinomatous component, or an otherwise squamous carcinoma with occasional intracytoplasmic mucin does not meet the diagnostic criteria of adenosquamous carcinoma.

*Adenoid basal carcinoma* is seen mostly in postmenopausal patients, particularly African–Americans. The carcinoma consists of lobules of wildly spaced nests of small uniform cells resembling those of a basal cell carcinoma. Peripheral palisading and central cystic formation are characteristic (Fig. 4.19). Pseudocysts and intraluminal hyaline materials seen in adenoid cystic carcinoma

**Fig. 4.19** Adenoid basal carcinoma. Note the wildly spaced nests of small uniform tumor cells, and peripheral palisading and central cystic formation (H.E. ×40)

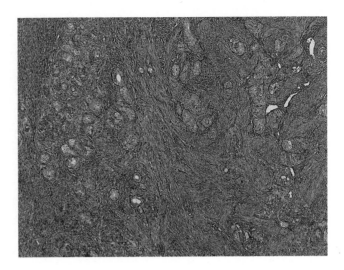

are not present in adenoid basal carcinoma. Benign adenoid basal hyperplasia is microscopic, noninvasive, and superficially located in connection with the surface epithelium.

*Mesonephric adenocarcinoma* arises from the embryonic remnant of mesonephric duct and frequently involves the deep lateral cervix. Histologically, the tumor has a ductal growth pattern, with tubular glands that are varying in size and lined by columnar cells. Intraluminal eosinophilic secretion is characteristic. Papillary, endometrioid, sex cord-like, and solid patterns are present focally or diffusely in some cases. The presence of adjacent mesonephric hyperplasia is a helpful hint for the diagnosis. Cytokeratin, EMA, calretinin, and particularly apical CD10 immunohistochemical positivity confirms the diagnosis. Clear cells with hobnailed nuclei are not features of mesonephric adenocarcinoma (see below).

*Clear cell and serous carcinomas* are high-grade adenocarcinomas that are essentially identical to those of the endometrium. Cervical clear cell carcinoma unrelated to DES exposure occurs in older patients, and those related to DES exposure are much younger, in their late 20s, and have a better survival. All histologic types of clear cell carcinoma can be seen, with tubocystic pattern being the most common. Cervical serous carcinoma can occur in patients younger than 40 years of age (Fig. 4.20), a patient group in

which primary endometrial serous carcinoma is exceedingly rare. P53 and p16 positivity are characteristic.

*Adenoid cystic carcinoma* consists of round to oval tumor nests of small basaloid cells of varying size with high N/C ratio. Palisading of tumor cells along the basement membrane is often found. Characteristic cribriforming due to the presence of pseudocysts/cylindrical hyaline basement membrane materials is diagnostic.

*Neuroendocrine carcinomas* include typical and atypical carcinoid tumors, and small and large cell neuroendocrine carcinomas. These tumors occur in a wide range of age, from 20 to 80 years. All have expression of one or more neuroendocrine (chromogranin, synaptophysin, CD56, and PGP 9.5) and epithelial markers by immunohistochemistry. Typical carcinoid has rare mitosis (less than 5/10 HPF), minimal nuclear atypia, and no necrosis. Atypical carcinoid has 5–10 mitosis/10 HPF, obvious nuclear atypia, and necrosis. Small cell neuroendocrine carcinoma resembles those of the lung: small anaplastic cells with scant cytoplasm, fine chromatin, and inconspicuous nucleoli along with nuclear molding and nuclear smudging (Fig. 4.21). Single to extensive tumor cell necrosis is common, so is lymphovascular invasion. Large cell neuroendocrine carcinoma is composed of medium to large, highly atypical cells with abundant cytoplasm and numerous mitoses

**Fig. 4.20** Cervical serous carcinoma (H.E. ×200)

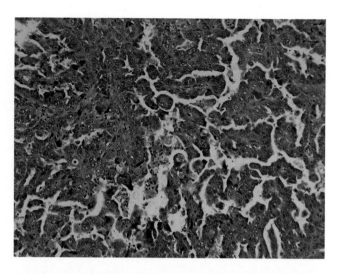

**Fig. 4.21** Small cell carcinoma of the cervix Note the presence of small anaplastic cells with scant cytoplasm, fine chromatin, and inconspicuous nucleoli along with nuclear molding (H.E. ×200)

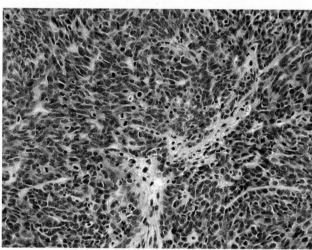

(>10/10 HPF). Geographic necrosis, peripheral nuclear palisading, and cytoplasmic granules are common findings. Both small and large cell neuroendocrine carcinomas are highly aggressive tumors and may be associated with cervical intraepithelial neoplasia, carcinoma in-site, or HPV positivity.

## 4.4 Cytology of Cervical Glandular Lesions

TBS recommends subclassifying atypical glandular cells (AGC) according to their origin: endocervical versus endometrial. If the origin cannot

be determined, the generic "glandular" terms should be used. Except for AGC of endometrial origin, TBS also recommends to further qualify AGC and AGC of endocervical origin (AEC) as "favor neoplastic" if deemed appropriate.

### 4.4.1 Atypical Glandular Cells, Endocervical Origin

AGC of endocervical origin is defined as endocervical cells displaying "nuclear atypia that exceeds obvious reactive or reparative changes but that lack unequivocal features of endocervical AIS or invasive adenocarcinoma." AEC is

**Fig. 4.22** Atypical glandular cells (AGC), endocervical origin. A cluster of endocervical cells with considerable nuclear crowding and overlapping. Individual cells demonstrate nuclear enlargement, increased N:C ratio, and hyperchromasia. Anisonucleosis is noted (ThinPrep, Papanicolaou, ×400)

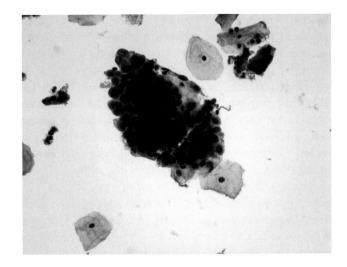

**Fig. 4.23** AGC, endocervical origin, favor neoplasia. Hyperchromatic crowded group of endocervical cells with marked nuclear crowding and overlapping. Features suggestive of feathering are noted in the upper portion of the cluster. Individual cells are markedly enlarged with hyperchromatic nuclei (SurePath, Papanicolaou, ×400)

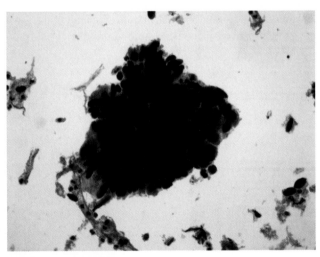

characterized by glandular cells occurring in sheets and strips, with considerable nuclear crowding and overlapping. Individual cells demonstrate nuclear enlargement up to 3–5× that of normal endocervical cells. There may be mild hyperchromasia, slight increase in N:C ratio, and mild degree of anisonucleosis (Fig. 4.22). Nucleoli, single or multiple, may be present and mitotic figures are rarely noted. Similar to ASC, not all of the criteria need to exist to arrive at an interpretation of ASC-US.

AEC favor neoplasia are often reserved for cases that resemble endocervical AIS or invasive carcinoma, but some salient features such as rosette formation, feathering, pseudostratification, or tumor diathesis are missing or poorly developed (Fig. 4.23). When compared to AEC-NOS, AEC-favor neoplasia displays more conspicuous nuclear crowding and overlapping, anisonucleosis, and higher N:C ratio.

Despite the name, majority of the AEC were found to have an underlying SIL on subsequent follow-up.

## 4.4.2 Endocervical Adenocarcinoma In Situ

A cytologic diagnosis of AIS often relies on the presence of characteristic architectural features. The neoplastic cells of AIS are often readily noticeable at low magnification because they appear as hyperchromatic crowded groups. In addition to small sheets and irregular groups, distinctive architectural features include feathering (nuclei protruding beyond the confines of the cells at the periphery of the clusters), rosette formation (two-dimensional clusters with cells arranged around a central lumen, with cytoplasm toward the center and nuclei at the periphery), pseudostratification (strips of neoplastic cells with nuclear crowding and loss of polarity), and acini formation (glandular structures within three-dimensional groups) (Figs. 4.24 and 4.25). Single cells are infrequent.

Individual cells often appear columnar with enlarged, elongated, and hyperchromatic nuclei. Anisonucleosis is usually absent or mild. Nucleoli are generally inconspicuous. Mitotic figures and apoptotic bodies are common and helpful to differentiate from benign lesions when present. There may be evidence of coexisting SIL.

In LBP, single intact cells are more readily identified. Individual groups tend to be smaller, denser, and more three-dimensional. Psuedostratification is prominent (Fig. 4.26). However, other architectural features, such as feathering and rosette formation, are less apparent.

It is important to note that the cytologic features of AIS just described are only pertinent to the classic variant, the most common type. Other variants such as intestinal, endometrioid, and clear cell carcinomas may demonstrate different morphologic features which can be interpreted as AGC-NOS, AGC-favor neoplasia, or even benign endometrial/endocervical cell groups.

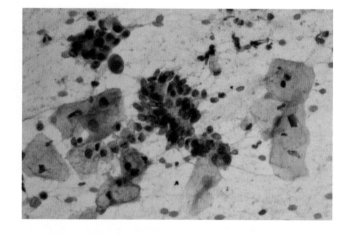

**Fig. 4.24** Adenocarcinoma in situ (AIS). Crowded group of columnar cells with elongated, hyperchromatic nuclei. At the periphery of the group, the nuclei protrude out without any cytoplasm – feathering (conventional preparation, Papanicolaou, ×400)

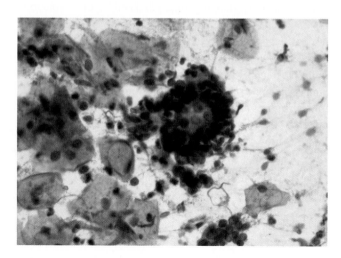

**Fig. 4.25** AIS. Three-dimensional crowded group of endocervical cells arranged in a glandular structure (conventional preparation, Papanicolaou, ×400)

**Fig. 4.26** AIS. Strips of endocervical cells with nuclear crowding and overlapping as well as loss of polarity (ThinPrep, Papanicolaou, ×400)

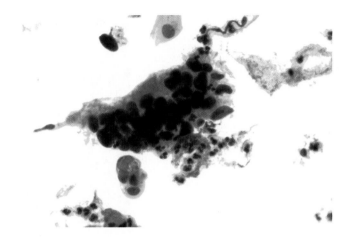

**Fig. 4.27** Endocervical adenocarcinoma. Loosely cohesive group of atypical glandular cells with high N:C ratio, hyperchromatic nuclei, and distinct nucleoli (conventional preparation, Papanicolaou, ×400)

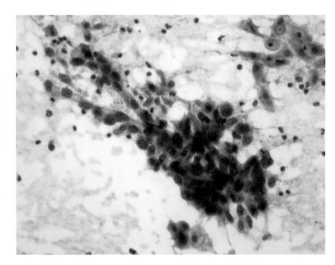

### 4.4.3  Endocervical Adenocarcinoma

Invasive endocervical adenocarcinoma is characterized by three-dimensional disorderly groups and clusters, often in a background of tumor diathesis. Glandular structures may be present. Single atypical cells are common. When the tumor is well differentiated, it may share cytologic features indistinguishable from those of AIS and individual cells often assume a columnar shape. It is important to remember that AIS may coexist with invasive adenocarcinoma; hence, cells from both lesions may be evident on the slide.

When the tumor becomes less differentiated, cytologic features of AIS will become ill defined and individual cells become round to oval. Nuclear enlargement, increased N:C ratio, anisonucleosis, coarsely granular chromatin, and macronucleoli are readily noted (Figs. 4.27 and 4.28). The amount of cytoplasm is variable but is generally more than that seen in endometrial adenocarcinoma. The cytoplasm often appears granular or finely vacuolated. Distinguishing the neoplastic cells of poorly differentiated endocervical adenocarcinoma from that of poorly differentiated endometrial adenocarcinoma and nonkeratinizing SCC may be difficult.

### 4.4.4  Mimics of Neoplastic Diseases

#### 4.4.4.1  Reactive Endocervical Cells

Reactive endocervical cells can demonstrate nuclear enlargement up to 3× that of a normal endocervical cell. Mild hyperchromasia may be

**Fig. 4.28** Endocervical adenocarcinoma. Several small clusters of glandular cells with marked nuclear crowding and overlapping. Many single atypical glandular cells are also noted. Individual cells often have a columnar appearance with vesicular chromatic and prominent nucleoli (SurePath, Papanicolaou, ×400)

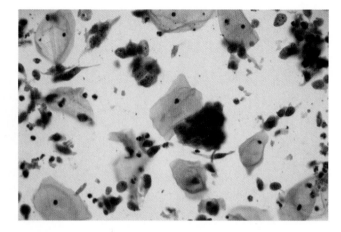

**Fig. 4.29** Reactive endocervical cells. Cluster of endocervical cells with minimal nuclear crowding and overlapping. Individual cells demonstrate nuclear enlargement, normal N:C ratio, and a small, distinct nucleoli (SurePath, Papanicolaou, ×400)

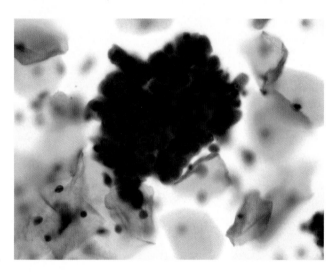

evident but the chromatin remains finely granular and evenly distributed. Nuclear outlines are smooth and round. Prominent single or multiple nucleoli are common (Fig. 4.29). Cytoplasmic inclusions containing neutrophils may be seen. There is minimal nuclear crowding and overlapping within the sheets and groups. These changes, often in the absence of an inflammatory background, can be seen in women wearing an intrauterine contraceptive device (IUD) because of the irritation of the endocervical canal caused by the string.

### 4.4.4.2 Tubal Metaplasia

Tubal metaplasia refers to the process in which endocervical epithelium is replaced by epithelium similar to that of the fallopian tube. On cytology, these cells are columnar in shape and arrange as crowded groups and strips with pseudostratification. There is considerable cellular pleomorphism. Individual nuclei tend to be round and oval with evenly distributed chromatin (Figs. 4.30 and 4.31). Because of the overcrowding and pseudostratification, tubal metaplastic cells are often classified as AGC or AIS. A definitive diagnosis of tubal metaplasia requires the identification of the cilia and/or terminal bars. In addition, AIS tends to have more elongated nuclei in contrast to the round to oval nuclei with tubal metaplasia. Hyperchromasia and increased N:C ratio are not helpful features because they can be seen in both tubal metaplasia and AIS.

**Fig. 4.30** Tubal metaplasia. Strips of endocervical cells with nuclear overlapping and crowding (ThinPrep, Papanicolaou, ×400)

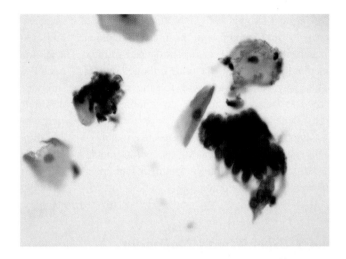

**Fig. 4.31** Tubal metaplasia. Crowded cluster of endocervical cells. Individual cells demonstrate nuclear enlargement and mild increase in N:C ratio. Ciliated endocervical cells often noted (*circle*) (ThinPrep, Papanicolaou, ×400)

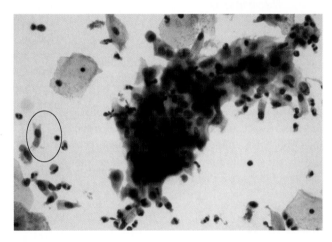

### 4.4.4.3  Microglandular Hyperplasia

MGH is usually associated with excess progesterone effects such as that of pregnancy and oral contraceptives. The cells of MGH demonstrate orangeophilic cytoplasm and pyknotic nuclei, resembling parakeratotic cells; they are often classified as atypical squamous cells.

### 4.4.4.4  Benign Glandular Cells Status Post-Hysterectomy

Benign glandular cells may be seen in 10% of patients who have undergone total hysterectomy. They resemble benign endocervical cells. They can be derived from vaginal adenosis, tubal prolapse, mesonephric duct remnants, vaginal endometriosis, and rectovaginal fistula.

### 4.4.4.5  Pregnancy-Related Changes

Arias-Stella reaction affects both endocervical and endometrial glandular cells as a result of increased levels of estrogen and progesterone. The cytologic finding consists of the presence of single or clusters of large cells, with a variable degree of pleomorphism and degenerative changes. Awareness of a history of pregnancy is important in order to avoid overinterpretation as adenocarcinoma.

Cervical stromal cells may undergo decidual changes in pregnant and postpartum women. The decidualized cells are about the size of intermediate squamous cells with enlarged nuclei. They may be mistaken as dysplastic squamous cells, especially when the decidualized cells show degenerative changes.

Cytotrophoblasts, resembling reactive squamous cells, and syncytial trophoblasts, as multinucleated giant cells, are rarely found in Pap specimens of pregnant women.

## 4.4.5 Other Primary Malignant Neoplasms

Primary cervical malignant neoplasms, other than squamous cell carcinomas and adenocarcinomas, are uncommon and may rarely be seen in gynecologic cytology. Only a few of these tumors may present characteristic features to allow a definitive diagnosis based on morphology alone. For the majority of these tumors, a definitive diagnosis is usually impossible because of limited sampling and morphologic overlap with other entities.

### 4.4.5.1 Sarcomas

Uterine sarcomas seldom exfoliate. In addition, their cytology varies depending on the histologic subtypes and the grade of the sarcomas. For example, the neoplastic cells of low-grade endometrial stromal sarcomas resemble those of normal endometrial stromal cells with minimal cytologic atypia. On the contrary, marked cytologic atypia is usually observed with leiomyosarcoma, high-grade endometrial stromal sarcomas, and malignant mixed Mullerian tumors (MMMT). The latter may demonstrate a biphasic pattern of carcinoma and sarcoma.

### 4.4.5.2 Melanoma

The cytology is similar to that occurring in other parts of the body. The typical presentation involves isolated and loosely cohesive large epithelioid and/or spindle-shaped cells with variable amount of cytoplasm, and round to oval nuclei with prominent nucleoli. Occasionally, spindle-shaped neoplastic cells can be seen. The differential diagnosis includes poorly differentiated carcinoma, lymphoma, and sarcoma. In addition, metastasis from an extra cervical melanoma should be ruled out.

### 4.4.5.3 Lymphoma

Both Hodgkin's and non-Hodgkin's lymphomas have been described in gynecologic cytology; however, the latter are more frequent. Non-Hodgkin's lymphomas typically present with a monotonous population of lymphocytes. The differential diagnosis includes follicular cervicitis, small cell carcinoma, and poorly differentiated carcinoma.

Follicular cervicitis is characterized by the presence of a heterogeneous population of lymphocytes with scattered intermixed plasma cells and tingible body macrophages (Fig. 4.32). The lymphocytes are usually dispersed in conventional preparation, but form loose clusters in LBP. It is important to recognize follicular cervicitis to avoid mistaking it as an HSIL, lymphoma, and small cell carcinoma. Both HSIL and small cell carcinoma display cohesive clusters and conspicuous nuclear pleomorphism. Lymphomas are characterized by the presence of a uniform population of lymphocytes. Except for HSIL, a known history of prior malignancy is often available since primary lymphoma or small cell carcinoma of the cervix is very rare.

### 4.4.5.4 Metastatic Tumors

Metastatic tumors of the uterine cervix also occur rarely. Knowledge of a prior malignancy and comparison with prior pathologic materials are helpful in arriving at the correct diagnosis (Figs. 4.33 and 4.34).

**Fig. 4.32** Follicular cervicitis. Clusters of mixed small and large lymphocytes are noted. A tingible body macrophage is present among the lymphocytes (ThinPrep, Papanicolaou, ×400)

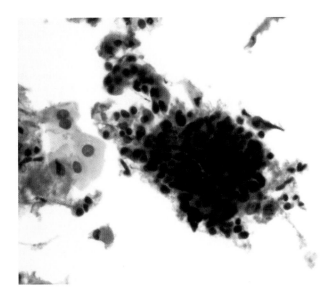

**Fig. 4.33** Melanoma, metastatic to cervix. Discohesive spindle cells with high N:C ratio and coarse chromatin (conventional preparation, Papanicolaou, ×400)

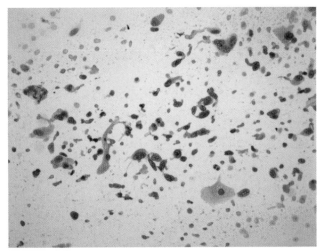

**Fig. 4.34** Colon carcinoma, metastatic to cervix. Loosely cohesive columnar glandular cells with high N:C ratio and pleomorphic nuclei (conventional preparation, Papanicolaou, ×400)

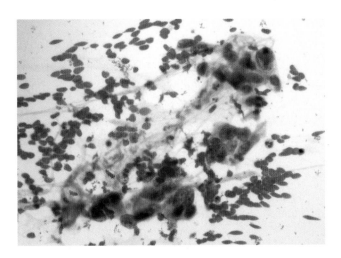

# Suggested Reading

Clement PB, Young RH. Atlas of Gynecologic Surgical Pathology. 2nd Edition. Saunders, Philadelphia, PA. 2008.

Diane S, Nayar R, Davey DD, and Wilbur DC. The Bethesda System for Reporting Cervical Cytology: Definitions, Criteria, and Explanatory Notes. 2nd Edition. Springer, New York. 2004.

Kurman R. Blaustein's Pathology of the Female Genital Tract. 5th Edition. Springer, New York. 2002.

Young RH, Clement PB. Endocervical adenocarcinoma and its variants: their morphology and differential diagnosis. Histopathology. 2002, 41: 185–207.

# Chapter 5
# Human Papillomavirus for Cervical Pathology

**Keywords** Human papillomavirus • Detection • Indication

## 5.1 Classification, Properties, and Viral Genome

Human papillomaviruses are oncoviruses with estimated 100 distinct genotypes and are related to skin and/or mucosal proliferative disorders. Certain types of human papillomavirus (HPV) affect specific tissue sites, for example, HPV 1, 2, 4, and 7 cause benign skin papillomas (wart) only. Related to gynecological cancers, approximately 30 types of anogenital HPV can be spread though sexual interactions and are further subclassified into high and low risk groups. Human cervical cancers including all squamous and most, if not all, adeno-carcinomas are induced by distinct groups of the high-risk genital HPVs including HPV 16, 18, 31, 33, 35, and 51. In contrast, low-risk HPV subtypes including HPV 6 and 11 are principally associated with anal-genital condyloma.

Body of evidence of molecular investigations has firmly established the molecular basis of cervical carcinogenesis induced by HPVs. Episomal or non-integrating HPV genome is associated, often in large quantity, with benign and preneoplastic conditions, such as condyloma and low-grade cervical intraepithelial neoplasia (CIN1). In contrast, integrated HPV into the host-cell genome is characteristic for high-grade intraepithelial neoplasias (CIN 2 and 3) and invasive cervical cancers. Such integration appears to be clonal, i.e., every tumor cell shares identical HPV integration site(s) in the genome.

HPVs are small, nonenveloped, double-stranded circular DNA of 8 kb with a limited cell tropism. Although encoding only eight genes, HPVs express two important regulatory proteins: E6 and E7. E6 and E7 are oncoproteins that can inactivate the host P53 and RB tumor suppressor genes through proteolytic degradation and protein sequestration, respectively, leading ultimately to cell proliferation. The integrated forms of high-risk HPVs, such as HPV 16 and 18, over-express their E6 and E7 proteins with high affinity of binding to p53 and RB, therefore promoting high grade transformation of cervical epithelial cells. Low-risk HPVs such as HPV 11 and 16 do not integrate into the host-cell genome, and produce only low-affinity E6 and E7, incapable of high-grade malignant transformation.

## 5.2 Natural History of HPV Infection

Infection with HPV is considered to be a necessary causal factor of essentially all invasive cervical cancers. While most men and women infected with HPV do not develop cancer, a subset will and may take decades to evolve. Certain cofactors appear important to facilitate the HPV induced carcinogenesis, including host immune status, early age at first intercourse, multiple sexual partners, smoking, nutritional status, parity, HLA types and coinfection with other virus such as HIV-1 and herpes simplex virus.

D. Chhieng and P. Hui (eds.), *Cytology and Surgical Pathology of Gynecologic Neoplasms*,
Current Clinical Pathology, DOI 10.1007/978-1-60761-164-6_5,
© Springer Science+Business Media, LLC 2011

Patients over 30 years of age with persistent high-risk HPV infection are at significantly increased risk for developing invasive cervical cancer. It is important to understand that HPV infection, particularly of the high-risk group, may have long-term consequences of cancer development later in adulthood. Current HPV vaccination may alter the natural course of the disease process, and long-term social and biomedical outcome of such general vaccination may not be fully appreciated until a decade or later.

## 5.3  Distribution of HPV in Cervical Lesions

HPV induced cervical intraepithelial lesions essentially start at the squamocolumnar junction in the transformation zone of the cervix. Not all HPV related lesions present as condyloma or low-grade lesions; high-grade lesions may appear at any point of the infection depending on HPV types and quantity. The presence of large amount of HPV in condyloma acuminatum coincides with the appearance of koilocytosis, usually present in the upper half of the infected epithelium. In contrast, in a high-grade cervical intraepithelial neoplasia or invasive cancer, integrated forms of HPV virus detectable by in-situ hybridization appear as single-cell nuclear positivity, due to low amount of integrated viral DNA.

## 5.4  Methods of Detection

Various molecular platforms have become available for the clinical detection and subtyping of HPV using both tissue and cytological specimens. Signal amplification assays (Digene hybrid capture 2 assay and Hologic invader displacement analysis), polymerase chain reaction, and in-situ hybridization are commonly employed methods. However, the latter two are not readily applicable to cytological fluid specimens.

Digene hybrid capture 2 (HCII) assay is FDA approved platform for clinical applications using cytological specimens (PAP smear), although competitive methods such as invader technology is comparable and just received the FDA approval. HCII employs a cocktail of specific RNA probes to detect HPV DNA released from a specimen. The HCII high-risk cocktail targets 13 high-risk HPVs (16, 18, 31, 35, 39, 45, 51, 52, 56, 58, 59, and 68). Specific hybrids formed between the probes and HPV DNA are captured onto solid surface in a microtiter well coated with specific antibodies for RNA-DNA hybrids. Alkaline phosphatase-linked antibodies recognize the immobilized RNA-DNA hybrids and then amplify the signals, which are eventually translated into measurable chemiluminescent signals created during substrate cleavage by the phosphatase enzyme. The end light emission is measured as relative light units (RLU). Specimens with RLU/CO (cutoff value) of more than 1.0 are considered positive for HPV infection.

Hologic Invader Technology employs isothermal signal amplification to detect the 13 high-risk HPV subtypes using three probe pools based on phylogenetic relatedness. It also incorporates an internal control for human alpha-actin to control for DNA quality and quantity. The invader technique appears comparable with the HCII, both have HPV16 and 18 genotyping capabilities.

## 5.5  Indications for HPV Testing

Early detection of cervical cancer has been clinically successful and cytological screening of Papanicolau smear has resulted in reduced incidence and mortality of cervical cancer. Now, HPV detection has been incorporated into the early screening and management programs in the USA.

Reflex HPV testing has been part of the clinical screening algorithm in women with equivocal cytology – atypical squamous cells of undetermined significance (ASCUS) in the past 10 years. As an interim recommendation by the American Cancer Society and the American College of

Obstetrics and Gynecology, a combined approach using both cytology and HPV testing has been endorsed for clinical practice in 2006. In underdeveloped countries where cytology is not readily available, HPV testing may offer the next best screening method for early detection and prevention of cervical cancer. More recently, it has been recommended that for women over 30 years of age, HPV viral testing should be the primary screening method in the USA (see Section 5.6.3).

Biopsy of the cervix is still the gold standard to document HPV related lesions including HPV infection (condyloma), preneoplastic conditions (CINs), and invasive cancers. Indications of colposcopy biopsy include abnormal PAP smears, persistent HPV infections, and unsatisfied PAP or HPV screening in patients with high risk.

## 5.6 Applications for HPV Testing in Cytology

The goal of applying HR HPV DNA testing in gynecologic cytology is to provide an objective mean to identify women who are at risk for developing cervical neoplasia. Currently, HR HPV DNA testing has been indicated for primary screening with Pap tests, triage of ASC-US or LSIL, and surveillance after treatment for CIN.

### 5.6.1 Triage of ASC-US and/or LSIL

ASC-US accounts for the majority of the abnormal Pap tests. About 30–40% of these cases will have an underlying CIN lesion on subsequent biopsy. However, immediate referral to colposcopy of all patients with an ASC-US interpretation would result in many unnecessary invasive procedures. Until a decade ago, repeat cytology was the standard practice for patient with an ASC-US interpretation. However, repeat cytology is inherently subjective and requires additional clinic visit.

Based on a cohort of almost 3,500 women, the ASCUS-LSIL Triage Study (ALTS) evaluated three strategies for managing women with

ASC-US: immediate colposcopy, HR HPV DNA testing, and repeat cytology. All three methods demonstrated similar sensitivity in detecting high lesions. However, only half of the women were referred to colposcopy based on HPV testing triage whereas two thirds of women were referred to colposcopy based on repeat cytology using ASC-US as cutoff. The latter depends on patient compliance with multiple follow up visit. Both HPV DNA testing and repeated cytology with ASC-US as cutoff demonstrated similar specificity (~60%). Other studies have reported similar findings. It is not surprising that the use of HPV DNA testing in triage of ASC-US has been incorporated in many guidelines for managing abnormal gynecologic cytology. According to the literature, HPV DNA detection rates in specimens with an ASC interpretation range from 31 to 66%.

Triage of LSIL using HPV DNA testing is less well established. The HPV detection rates in specimens with LSIL interpretation range from 60 to 85%, significantly higher than that of ASC-US interpretation. According to the ALTS study, the specificity of reflex HPV DNA testing for detecting CIN 2+ was 16 and 30% in women younger than 29 with a LSIL cytologic interpretation and those 29 or older, respectively. Therefore, the current guidelines do not recommend reflex HPV DNA testing for the triage of LSIL.

### 5.6.2 Surveillance After Treatment of CIN

About 10% (0–36%) of women who are treated for CIN recur within the first 2 years; the risk of recurrence increases with age. Therefore, women treated for CIN should be followed up regularly. The sensitivity of HPV DNA testing in predicting short term treatment failure is about 95%, significantly higher than that of follow up cytology or positive histologic surgical margins with comparable specificity with all three methods. It has been recommended that women treated for CIN 2+ should have either consecutive Pap tests at 4–6 months interval or a single HPV DNA testing at least 6 months posttreatment. When there are either three consecutive negative Pap tests or a single negative HPV DNA testing, patients can return to the routine screening schedule.

### 5.6.3 Primary Screening

Several North American and Western European studies have demonstrated that high risk HPV DNA testing, as a primary screening test, has a higher sensitivity (25–35% higher) and a higher negative predictive value for detecting CIN 2+ lesions when compared to routine Pap tests. However, HPV testing has a lower specificity (10–15%) lower and a lower positive predictive value than routine Pap tests, resulting in increase referral to colposcopy. These can be attributed to the high prevalence of transient HPV infection in women in their late teens and early 20s. As a result, in United States, the FDA has approved the use of high risk HPV DNA testing in conjunction with routine cervical cytology screening in women age 30 years or older. Table 5.1 summarizes the recommended patients' management for various combinations of cytologic findings and HPV status. For a combined negative cytology and HPV test, the negative predictive value in predicting of developing a CIN 3+ over a 5-year period is 99.9%, i.e. only 9 per 10,000 will develop CIN 3+ over a 5-year period in the presence of a combined negative cytology and HPV test. Therefore, for women with combined negative results, the recommended screening interval is 3 years.

The use of HPV DNA testing as the sole primary screening method for cervical cancer offer several advantages: the test is highly sensitive and more objective, the assay can be automated, and the need of cytology is reduced. However, it is not currently recommended because HPV screening at a young age is not cost-efficient as a result of high prevalence of transient HPV infection. In addition, primary HPV screening demonstrates lower specificity and positive predictive value in predicting high grade CIN.

### 5.6.4 HPV Genotyping

Among the high risk HPV types, HPV 16 and 18 are responsible for approximately 70% of cervical cancers. It has been shown that the 10-year cumulative risk of detecting CIN 3+ was 17% and 13% for women positive for HPV 16 and HPV 18, respectively, whereas the 10 year cumulative risk of detecting CIN 3+ was 3% for women positive for high risk HPV, but negative for HPV 16 and 18. The current guidelines recommend women who have negative cytology, but positive HPV test result should be tested for HPV 16 and 18. If the patient were tested positive for either 16 or 18, she would be referred for immediate colposcopy. If the patient were negative for 16 and 18, she could be followed with repeat cytology and HPV DNA testing in 1 year.

**Table 5.1** Recommendation for various combination of HPV and cytology result for women undergoing HPV cotesting

| HPV result | Cytology result | Risk of CIN 3 or above | Suggested management |
|---|---|---|---|
| Negative | Negative | <0.1% | Repeat cytology alone in 1–2 year Cytology + HR HPV every 3 years |
| Positive | Negative | 2–10% | Rescreening in a year Genotyping for HPV 16 and 18 |
| Negative | ASC, ASC-H, LSIL, AEC, & AGC | 2–10% | Rescreening in a year |
| Positive | ASC, ASC-H, LSIL, AEC, & AGC | >10% | Immediate colposcopy |
| Positive/negative | HSIL | >40% | Immediate colposcopy |

## Suggested Reading

Astbury K, Turner MJ. Human papillomavirus vaccination in the prevention of cervical neoplasia. Int J Gynecol Cancer. 2009;19(9):1610–3.

Cuzick J, et al: Overview of human papillomavirus-based and other novel options for cervical cancer screening in developed and developing countries. Vaccine. 2008;26(10):K29–41.

Lizano M, et al: HPV-related carcinogenesis: basic concepts, viral types and variants. Arch Med Res. 2009;40(6):428–34.

Meijer CJ, Snijders PJ, Castle PE. Clinical utility of HPV genotyping. Gynecol Oncol. 2006;103(1): 12–7.

Zaravinos A, et al: Molecular detection methods of human papillomavirus (HPV). Int J Biol Markers. 2009;24(4):215–22.

# Chapter 6
# Endometrial Epithelial Neoplasms

**Keywords** Endometrium • Hyperplasia • Carcinoma

## 6.1 General Classification of Uterine Corpus Neoplasms

Nonneoplastic lesions of the endometrium encompass a broad spectrum of epithelial alternations ranging from metaplasia, hormonal-related changes, inflammatory processes, reparative conditions, endometrial polyps and gestational alterations. Many of these conditions can mimic various malignant or pre-malignancy lesions of the endometrium, particularly when present in a small biopsy or curettage specimen. Endometrial hyperplasia and atypical hyperplasia are preneoplastic conditions that precede to the most common endometrioid adenocarcinoma (Type 1 endometrial cancer). Serous and clear-cell carcinomas (Type 2 endometrial cancer) are high-grade carcinomas by definition and account for about 10–15% of endometrial malignancy. Mucinous carcinomas are diagnosed based on varying percentages of mucinous component present in the tumor, and is graded and treated as endometrioid carcinoma. Other histological types are rare, including squamous cell carcinoma, transitional cell carcinoma, undifferentiated carcinomas (small cell and non-small cell), and finally various mixed carcinomas when individual mixed component constitutes at least 10% of the entire tumor.

## 6.2 Benign Tumors and Tumor-Like Conditions

*Endometrial polyp* is a common lesion found in about 24% of women. It may be sessile or pedunculated, single or multiple with sizes from less than 1 cm to filling up the entire endometrial cavity. Polyps are generally classified into hyperplastic, atrophic, or functional types based on the status of glandular epithelium. The stromal component is generally fibrotic with thickened vasculatures. Smooth muscle fibers can be found sparsely in some endometrial polyps. When intact, recognition of the polyp is straightforward. Most polyps are fragmented in small biopsy or curettage specimens (Fig. 6.1). In a background of normal appearing endometrium, the presence of tissue fragments with fibrotic stroma, thickened vasculatures, crowded and/or irregular endometrial glands signifies the presence of an endometrial polyp. Endometrial polyps can be associated with atypical hyperplasia, endometrioid adenocarcinoma and importantly minimal uterine serous carcinoma. The presence of scattered plasma cells is common and should not be interpreted as chronic endometritis.

*Adenomatoid tumor* is benign tumors of the mesothelial origin. These are solitary, less well-defined lesions, involving subserosa or myometrium. The lesion consists of proliferation of glands, tubules, cystic spaces, or solid tumor nests (Fig. 6.2). The lining cells are round, or cuboidal, or flattened with eosinophilic cytoplasm of mesothelial nature. The present

D. Chhieng and P. Hui (eds.), *Cytology and Surgical Pathology of Gynecologic Neoplasms*, Current Clinical Pathology, DOI 10.1007/978-1-60761-164-6_6, © Springer Science+Business Media, LLC 2011

**Fig. 6.1** Endometrial polyp. Note the fibrotic stroma, thickened vasculatures, and irregular glands (H.E. ×40)

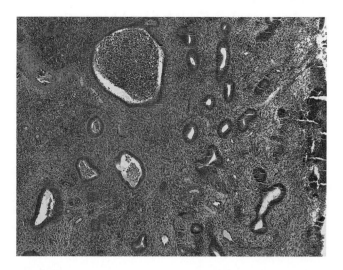

**Fig. 6.2** Adenomatoid tumor. The tumor consists of lobules of tubular to cystic spaces lined by flattened mesothelial cells (H.E. ×40)

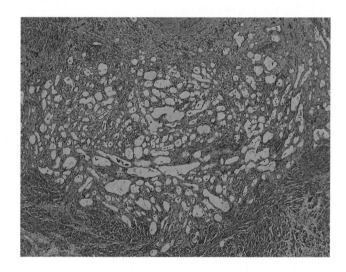

intraglandular cytoplasmic bridging is a helpful hint to the diagnosis. The surrounding myometrial smooth-muscle cells are frequently hyperplastic and nodular. The tumor cells are typically positive for cytokeratin, vimentin, WT-1, and calretinin.

Teratoma, ectopic tissue (brain or cartilage), benign papillary serous tumor, postoperative spindle-cell nodule, and lymphoma-like lesions are among rare tumor-like conditions.

Metaplastic changes of the endometrium are frequent findings that may mimic a neoplastic or pre-neoplastic process. Eosinophilic and papillary syncytial metaplasia are often associated with breakdown endometrium, particularly abnormal bleeding. Squamous metaplasia can be seen in both benign endometrium, endometrioid carcinoma and its precursor – endometrial hyperplasia. Tubal or ciliate metaplasia has tubal-type epithelium and is often found in normal proliferative endometrium or in isolated glands of atrophic endometrium. Clear-cell metaplasia involves endometrial glands that have clear cytoplasm containing glycogen. Secretory changes can superimpose on either hyperplasia or carcinoma with columnar cells having sub- or supranuclear

**Fig. 6.3** Endometrial mucinous change with increased glandular complexity (H.E. ×100)

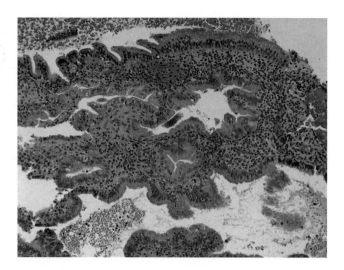

**Fig. 6.4** Endometrial mucinous change with marked glandular complexity and cytological atypia (H.E. ×200)

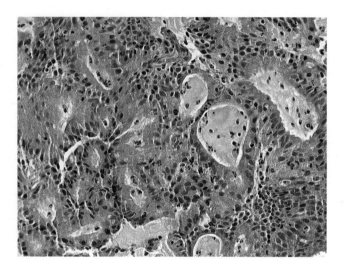

vacuoles, simulating early secretory endometrial glands. Mucinous changes are almost always of endocervical type and can be seen in both benign and malignant conditions. Three types of mucinous changes have been characterized with corresponding clinical implications. Simple, nonatypical mucinous changes are benign and inconsequential. Complex mucinous changes including microglandular and cribriform patterns without cytological atypia should prompt additional sampling or hysterectomy to rule out well-differentiated endometrioid carcinoma (Fig. 6.3). Highly complex mucinous proliferation with

cribriform and branching villous epithelium and cytological atypia is almost always associated with well-differentiated adeno carcinoma (Fig. 6.4).

## 6.3 Endometrial Hyperplasia

Endometrial hyperplasia is defined as disproportionate glandular proliferation resulting in an abnormal gland/stroma ratio. It is further divided into typical and atypical forms based on the absence or presence of cytological atypia in the glandular component. Four subcategories are conventionally diagnosed: simple hyperplasia, complex hyperplasia, atypical simple hyperplasia, and atypical complex hyperplasia. It should be noted that separation of atypical hyperplasia from those of nonatypical ones is of clinical relevance for subsequent patient management.

Hyperplasia without atypia is characterized by diffuse glandular proliferation of nonatypical epithelium with either balanced gland/stroma ratio (simple hyperplasia, Fig. 6.5), or marked increase gland/stroma ratio (complex hyperplasia, Fig. 6.6). The glands are abnormal in shape (cystic, pouching and branching) and sizes.

The glandular epithelium is columnar and pseudostratified. Mitotic activity is variable. The stroma in simple hyperplasia is abundant and densely packed with plump spindle cells. The stromal component is diminished in complex hyperplasia leading to more glandular crowding with back-to-back configuration. Generally speaking, glandular abnormalities are more pronounced in a complex than a simple hyperplasia. Lesser degree proliferative lesions such as disordered proliferation endometrium show isolated glandular abnormalities scattered within otherwise normal proliferative endometrium. However, hyperplasia can be regional in some cases.

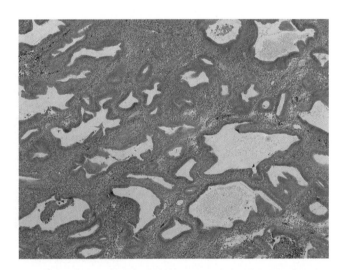

**Fig. 6.5** Simple endometrial hyperplasia. Note relatively balanced glandular and stromal components (H.E. ×40)

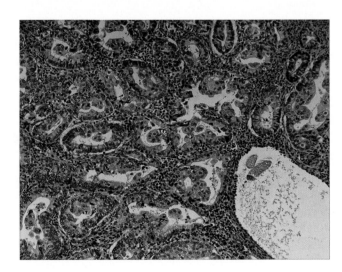

**Fig. 6.6** Atypical complex endometrial hyperplasia. Note the marked increase gland/stroma ratio and abnormal glandular shape (cystic, pouching, and branching) and sizes (H.E. ×100)

**Fig. 6.7** Cytological atypia of atypical hyperplasia. Note the nuclear rounding, enlargement, stratification, and loss of polarity (H.E. ×400)

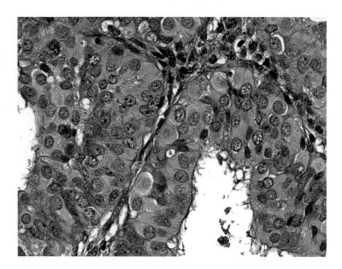

Atypicality of hyperplasia is defined by the nuclear alterations of the glandular epithelium. Nuclear rounding, enlargement, variation in size, stratification and loss of polarity are diagnostic features (Fig. 6.7). Nuclear chromatin shows clumping and nuclear membrane may be thickened. In some atypical cells, the nuclei may have a vesicular chromatin pattern with condensation along the nuclear membrane. The nuclear atypia should be present in significant number or clusters of cells of the involved glands. Occasional atypical cells should be ignored, and in practice, a comparison with adjacent normal endometrial glands is helpful to confirm the presence of nuclear atypicality. Grading of the cytological atypia is subjective and generally not clinically useful, unless the presence of grade 3 nuclei, which may indicate the presence of intraepithelial serous carcinoma or endometrial intraepithelial carcinoma (EIC).

Endometrial intraepithelial neoplasia (EIN) classification of precursor lesions of endometrial carcinoma has been recently advocated. The classification is based on the combination of architecture, cytological features, size of the lesion, exclusion of benign mimics, and exclusion of carcinoma. The system appears to have better reproducibility in the classification of preneoplastic lesions and in-situ carcinoma.

Separation of a highly atypical complex hyperplasia from a well differentiated endometrioid carcinoma can be difficult and subjective, particularly in a small biopsy or curettage. However, this may not be clinically important as both require hysterectomy in general. Three histological findings indicate an invasive carcinoma: (1) an altered stroma among atypical endometrial glands. Desmoplastic stroma with fibroblasts or myofibroblasts that rigidly exist between the glands indicates an invasive carcinoma. Disappearance of normal endometrial stromal cells with replacement by aggregates of foamy macrophages or eosinophilic collagen deposition also suggests stromal invasion (Fig. 6.8); (2) confluent expansion of atypical glands without intervening stromal component. Glands are back-to-back without stroma in between, or merging into each other to from complex labyrinth or cribriform patterns (Fig. 6.9); (3) expansile glands with complex papillation (Fig. 6.10). The presence of the above three alterations must exceed 2 mm$^2$ in a single focus to qualify a diagnosis of adenocarcinoma.

## 6.4 Endometrial Carcinomas

Endometrial carcinoma is the most common cancer of the female genital tract. In the USA, in 2008, some 40,000 new cases were diagnosed and 7,000 or so died of the disease. Long term estrogen overload through obesity, hormone replacement, oral contraceptives, and smoking is significantly associated with the most common, endometrioid adenocarcinoma (Type 1

**Fig. 6.8** Endometrioid
adenocarcinoma. Note the
replacement of endometrial
stroma with think strands of
wavy collagen (H.E. ×200)

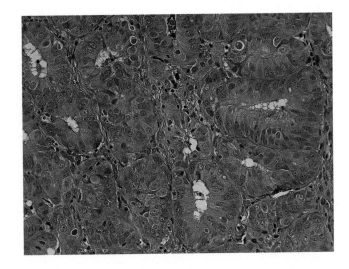

**Fig. 6.9** Endometrioid
adenocarcinoma. Note the
disappearance of stroma and
cribriforming of the glands
(H.E. ×100)

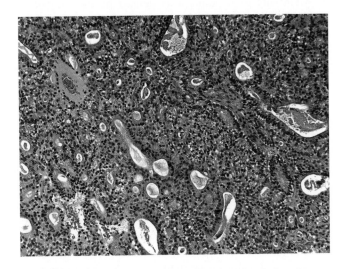

**Fig. 6.10** Endometrioid
adenocarcinoma with complex
papillation and an expansile
growth (H.E. ×100)

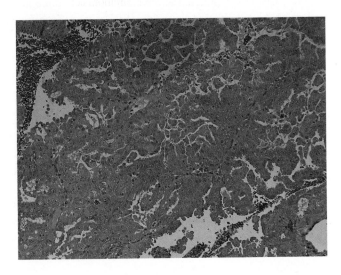

endometrial cancer) and its related precursor – endometrial hyperplasia. Subsets of endometrial cancers (10–15%) are serous and clear-cell carcinomas (Type 2 endometrial cancer). These tumors are high grade by definition and primarily found in postmenopausal patients. Classifications of malignant epithelial tumors are summarized in Table 6.1.

*Endometrioid carcinoma*, in its pure form, represents 60% of all uterine cancers. Over 20% are mixed with other carcinomatous components. Most cases occur in postmenopausal patients with vaginal bleeding. Single to multiple polypoid masses or diffuse endometrial involvement can be seen. Histologically, the tumor has a columnar epithelial proliferation in glandular patterns of various sizes and shapes, generally resembling proliferative endometrial glands (Fig. 6.11). Branching, papillary, or cribriform patterns are common. Percentage of the solid glandular growth dictates the histological grade (FIGO grade) of an endometrioid adenocarcinoma: 5% or less solid glandular component in FIGO grade 1, >5–50% in grade 2; and >50% in grade 3 (Figs. 6.11–6.13). Cytological atypia is present in all, but the degrees vary significantly from case to case. Some clinical practice requires reporting of the nuclear grade of an endometrioid carcinoma. A tumor with nuclear grade 1 consists of relatively uniform tumor cells with moderate nuclear enlargement, finely dispersed chromatin, and inconspicuous or small nucleoli (Fig. 6.14). Nuclear grade 2 indicates significant enlargement of tumor cells with obvious nuclear

**Table 6.1** Classifications of malignant epithelial tumors of endometrium

| Major heading | Subtype or variant | | | |
|---|---|---|---|---|
| Endometrioid | Conventional | | | |
| | Secretory | | | |
| | Villoglandular | | | |
| | Microglandular | | | |
| | Sertoliform | | | |
| | Ciliated | | | |
| | Papillary | | | |
| Serous | | | | |
| Clear cell | | | | |
| Mucinous | | 1 | | |
| Squamous | | | | |
| Transitional | | | | |
| Poorly differentiated | Lymphoepitheliomatous | Hepatoid | Giant cell | With trophoblastic differentiation |
| Undifferentiated | Large cell | Small cell | | |
| Mixed carcinomas | | | | |

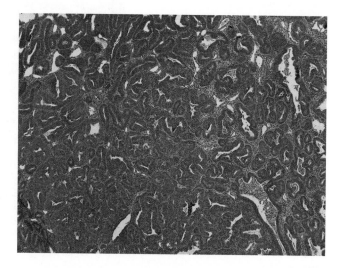

**Fig. 6.11** FIGO grade 1 endometrioid adenocarcinoma (H.E. ×40)

**Fig. 6.12** FIGO grade 2
endometrioid adenocarcinoma
(H.E. ×40)

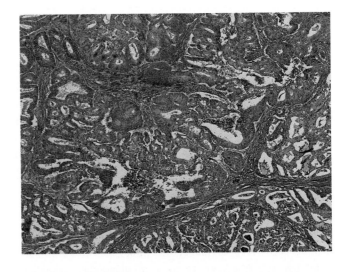

**Fig. 6.13** FIGO grade 3
endometrioid adenocarcinoma
(H.E. ×40)

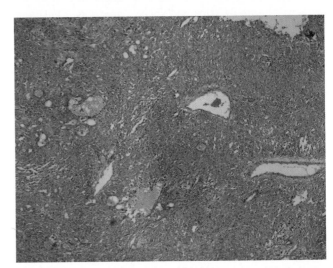

**Fig. 6.14** Nuclear grade 1
endometrioid adenocarcinoma
(H.E. ×200)

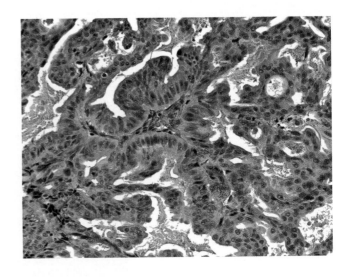

size variation and prominent nucleoli. Tumor cells of grade 3 nuclei show markedly nuclear enlargement, nuclear pleomorphism with three to four times size variation, large prominent nucleoli, marked hyperchromasia or coarse chromatin, and brisk mitotic figures with frequent abnormal mitosis (Fig. 6.15). The nuclear grades are generally parallel to the histological grades. However, in some cases, histological grade 1 or 2 tumor with grade 3 nuclear atypia, the FIGO grade should be up-scaled to 2 or 3, respectively. Endometrioid adenocarcinoma with squamous differentiation contains squamous elements of either matured (squamous morules to overt keratinization) or immature type (squamous metaplasia to squamous carcinomatous changes, Fig. 6.16). It is important that the grading of the tumor is based solely on the glandular component for both FIGO and nuclear grading.

There are several variants of endometrioid adenocarcinomas. Secretory carcinoma consists of tumor cells with subnuclear and/or supranuclear vacuolation. Ciliated-cell carcinoma shows extensive ciliated glandular cells involving at least 75% of the entire lesion. The villoglandular variant is diagnosed when the tumor consists of

**Fig. 6.15** Nuclear grade 3 endometrioid adenocarcinoma (H.E. ×200)

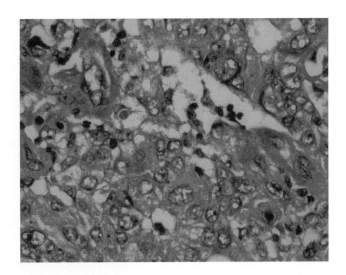

**Fig. 6.16** Endometrioid adenocarcinoma with marked squamous differentiation (H.E. ×200)

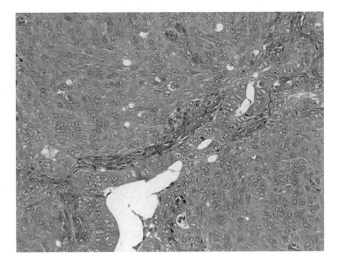

slender, delicate papillary fronts with thin or minimal stroma (Fig. 6.17). Secretory, ciliated, and villoglandular variants are almost always well differentiated with low nuclear grade. However, all can be associated with underlying myoinvasive conventional endometrioid carcinoma components. Papillary endometrioid carcinoma has hierarchical papillary branching simulating a serous carcinoma at low power, but the tumor cells are well differentiated with low nuclear grade (Fig. 6.18). Biopsy or curettage diagnosis of a microglandular endometrial carcinoma can be difficult due to its histological patterns simulating microglandular hyperplasia of the endocervix (Fig. 6.14).

*Mucinous carcinoma* is diagnosed when a significant portion (50–90%) of the tumor shows cytoplasmic mucin production. The majority consist of endocervical type mucinous cells arranged in glandular, cribriforming, villoglandular, and microglandular growth patterns (Fig. 6.19). Grading, treatment, and prognosis of mucinous carcinoma are similar to those of the conventional endometrioid carcinoma.

*Squamous cell carcinoma* is very rare and diagnosis of such follows the strict criteria including the absence of connection to cervical squamous epithelium, the absence of any glandular component, and the absence of cervical invasive squamous carcinoma. The histo-

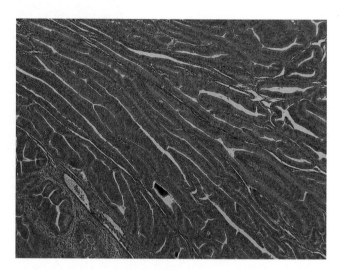

**Fig. 6.17** Villoglandular endometrioid adenocarcinoma (H.E. ×40)

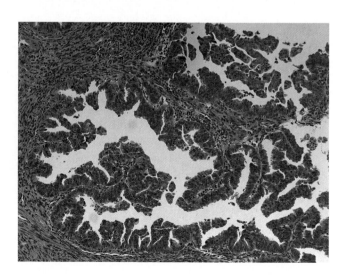

**Fig. 6.18** Papillary endometrioid adenocarcinoma (H.E. ×100)

**Fig. 6.19** Mucinous adenocarcinoma. Note the presence of obvious mucinous production in most of the tumor cells (H.E. ×100)

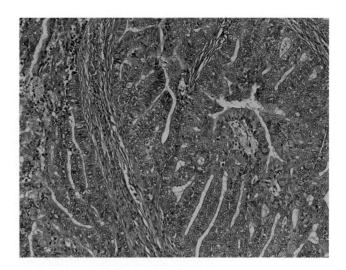

logical grades can range from well differentiated to poorly differentiated squamous cell carcinoma.

*Serous carcinoma (USC)* is a major histological subtype of the type 2 endometrial cancer, occurring almost always in a postmenopausal woman. Although representing 10% of all endometrial cancers, USC causes a disproportionate 50% of endometrial cancer deaths. Clinically USC is a high-grade malignancy and associated with tendency of deep myometrial invasion, high frequency of metastasis and unfavorable prognosis. Although its gross appearance is indistinguishable from endometrioid adenocarcinoma, USC has unique histological and cytological characteristics. The tumor consists of complex growth of short blunt cellular papillae with minimal stroma. The epithelium is composed of stratified tumor cells with secondary stroma-less papillae or cellular buds, frequently detached and free floating (Fig. 6.20a). Less common growth patterns of USC include elongated slit-like glandular spaces and solid sheet. Psammoma bodies are present in less than half of the cases; however, they are not diagnostically specific. The cytological features of USC are high grade by definition. The tumor cells show marked nuclear pleomorphism, nuclear megaly, and hyperchromasia. Macronucleoli are characteristic and often cherry-red in color with a perinucleolar halo. Mitotic figures are numerous and atypical forms are common (Fig. 6.20b). Bizarre nuclei, multinucleation, and hobnailing cells can be seen. Minimal uterine serous carcinoma has been proposed to include some early serous lesions, including endometrial intraepithelial serous carcinoma (formerly endometrial intraepithelial carcinoma) and superficial invasive serous carcinoma (stromal invasion of less than 1 cm). They are frequently associated with an endometrial polyp and many arise from it (Fig. 6.21). Recognition of minimal uterine serous carcinoma is clinically relevant as near half of the cases present with extrauterine tumors through transtubal spreading. Immunohistochemically, the tumor cells of USC are strongly and diffusely positive for P53, P16, and mib-1. ER and PR are usually negative or weakly patchy positive. WT-1 nuclear staining can be seen in a subset of the tumor and is not a reliable marker for separating from an ovarian primary serous carcinoma. USC should be separated from villoglandular and papillary endometrioid carcinomas. Filiform villous papillae are distinct features of villoglandular carcinoma. Both villoglandular and papillary endometrial carcinomas have single layer of low-grade tumor cells and are negative for P53 and P16 with low Mib-1 activity. Microglandular endometrioid carcinoma can be separated from USC by its typical cribriform glands and generally low nuclear grades, rather than slit-like growth pattern and high nuclear grade in USC. Over 1/3

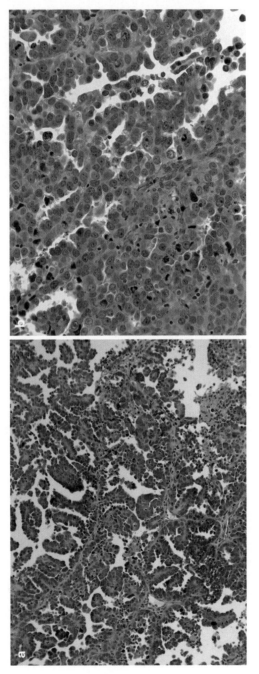

**Fig. 6.20** (**a, b**) Endometrial serous carcinoma. The tumor has a complex growth of short blunt cellular papillae with minimal stroma and stratified tumor cells with secondary stroma-less papillae or cellular buds, frequently detached and free floating (**a**, H.E. ×100). The tumor cells show grade 3 nuclear atypia and are highly mitotically active with frequent atypical forms (**b**, H.E. ×200)

**Fig. 6.21** Minimal serous carcinoma involving an endometrial polyp. Such early serous carcinoma may very subtle (H.E. ×20)

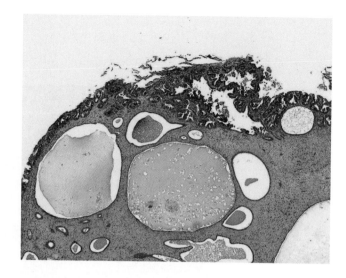

of USC are mixed carcinomas with endometrioid or clear-cell carcinoma as most common partners.

*Clear cell carcinoma (CCC)* is another type 2 endometrial carcinoma and represents up to 3% of all endometrial cancers. The most common histological pattern is tubocystic with high-grade tumor cells that have clear cytoplasm and typical hobnailed nuclei (Fig. 6.22a). Cells with abundant oxyphilic cytoplasm or flattened, small size clear cells are focally found as well. Short blunt papillae with eosinophilic hyalinized stroma are characteristic (Fig. 6.22b). Psammoma bodies are occasionally seen. The tumors have high level of mib-1 positivity with p16 expression in half of the cases and negative p53 staining in general.

Rare endometrial tumor types include transitional cell carcinoma, giant cell carcinoma, lymphoepitheliomatous carcinoma, hepatoid carcinoma, and poorly differentiated carcinoma

with trophoblastic differentiation. Undifferentiated carcinomas show no evidence of lineage differentiation and may be subtyped into non-small cell carcinoma and small-cell carcinoma. Most of the small-cell carcinomas are neuroendocrine in nature and highly aggressive.

Mixed carcinomas are not uncommon and any combinations of two carcinomatous components with at least 10% of each are required for the diagnosis. The common combinations include mixed endometrioid and mucinous carcinoma, and mixed endometrioid and serous carcinoma (Fig. 6.23).

## 6.5 Cytology

Table 6.2 summarizes the nomenclature used for describing the finding of endometrial cells in gynecologic cytology.

**Table 6.2** Comparison of reporting systems for endometrial cells

| Cytologic findings | TBS 2001 | ECTP 2007 | BSCC 2008 | AMBS 2004 |
|---|---|---|---|---|
| Benign EM cells <40 years | No need to report | No need to report | No need to report | No need to report |
| Benign EM cells ≥40 years | Report under the category of "Other" | EM cells in a postmenopausal woman | Negative, report presence of EM cells | Should not be reported |
| Atypical endometrial cells | Atypical endometrial cells | AGC, endometrial origin | ? Glandular neoplasia | AGC-US, Possible high grade glandular lesion |
| Endometrial adenocarcinoma | Adenocarcinoma, endometrial | Endometrial adenocarcinoma | Glandular neoplasia | Adenocarcinoma, endometrial |

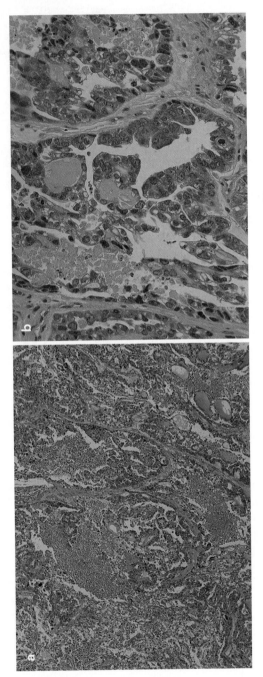

**Fig. 6.22** Clear-cell carcinoma of the endometrium. Low power view (**a**, H.E. ×40) and high power view (**b**, H.E. ×200)

**Fig. 6.23** Mixed serous and endometrioid carcinoma. Upper left serous carcinoma and lower right endometrioid component (H.E. ×100)

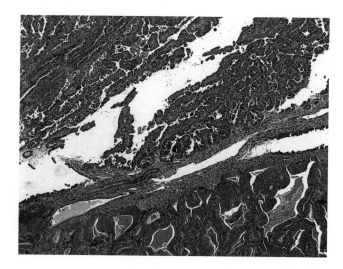

### 6.5.1 Atypical Glandular Cells, Endometrial Origin

AGC, endometrial origin (AMC) is characterized by small tight groups of 5–10 cells. Individual cells resemble normal endometrial glandular cells except with slightly enlarged nuclei (Figs. 6.24 and 6.25). Nucleoli may be present, especially with LBP. Cytoplasmic vacuoles are occasionally noted. As mentioned earlier, TBS does not recommend qualifying AMC because of lack of reproducible criteria.

### 6.5.2 Endometrial Adenocarcinoma

Exfoliated endometrial adenocarcinomas usually demonstrate few atypical cells. The tumor cells usually appear as small, tightly packed, three-dimensional groups, and occasionally isolated cells. The appearance of individual neoplastic cells depends on the degree of differentiation. For well-differentiated adenocarcinoma, the nuclei are only slightly enlarged when compared to their benign counterpart, often with inconspicuous nucleoli. The nuclei become larger with more prominent nucleoli when tumors become less differentiated. Cytoplasm is scanty, sometimes vacuolated with or without intracytoplasmic neutrophils (Figs. 6.26 and 6.27). Varying degree of degenerative changes can be seen. The background is sometimes described as watery and finely granular.

Direct sampling of endometrial adenocarcinoma that extends into the endocervical canal demonstrates quite different cytology. The cells often assume a columnar appearance with pseudostratification, similar to that of endocervical adenocarcinoma (Figs. 6.28 and 6.29).

Once a diagnosis of adenocarcinoma is made on Pap slide, the major differential diagnosis would be between endocervical and endometrial origin. Table 6.3 summarizes the cytologic differences between these two adenocarcinomas.

### 6.5.3 Gynecologic Cytology and the Detection of Endometrial Hyperplasia and Malignancy

Unlike their cervical counterpart, gynecology cytology has not been very successful as a screening tool for endometrial carcinoma and its precursor; up to 50% of endometrial carcinomas are missed during routine screening, often as a result of sampling error. Even when endometrial cells are identified, they often lack cytologic atypia.

Several cytologic findings have been reported to be associated with endometrial carcinomas and hyperplasias; high maturation index in postmenopausal women, abundant histiocytes, abnormal shedding of benign-appearing endometrial

**Fig. 6.24** AGC, endometrial origin. Small group of endometrial cells with enlarged, hyperchromatic nuclei, and vacuolated cytoplasm. Subsequent endometrial biopsy revealed chronic endometritis (ThinPrep, Papanicolaou, ×400)

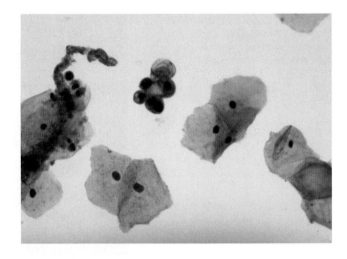

**Fig. 6.25** AGC, endometrial origin. Three-dimensional, tight group of endometrial with slightly enlarged nuclei. Subsequent endometrial sampling revealed a well differentiated endometrial carcinoma (conventional preparation, Papanicolaou, ×400)

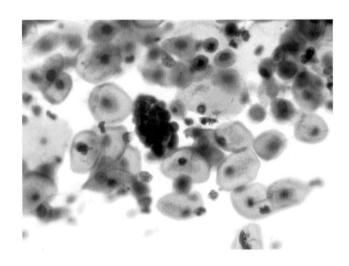

**Fig. 6.26** Endometrial adenocarcinoma, exfoliated. Small tight cluster of glandular cells with small amount of cytoplasm and high N:C ratio. Some cells possess cytoplasmic vacuoles. The nuclei are hyperchromatic (SurePath, Papanicolaou, ×400)

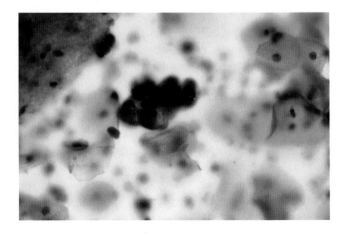

**Fig. 6.27** Endometrial adenocarcinoma, exfoliated. Small tight cluster of glandular cells. Intracytoplasmic vacuoles containing neutrophils is a frequent feature of endometrial adenocarcinoma. Endometrial adenocarcinoma, exfoliated (SurePath, Papanicolaou, ×400)

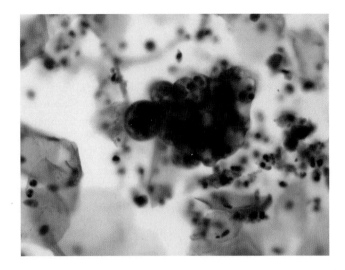

**Fig. 6.28** Endometrial adenocarcinoma, extension to endocervical canal. Crowded strip of columnar to low cuboidal cells with loss of polarity and nuclear crowding (conventional preparation, Papanicolaou, ×400)

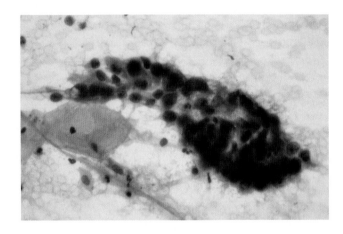

**Fig. 6.29** Endometrial adeno carcinoma, extension to endocervical canal. Sheets of atypical glandular cells with marked nuclear enlargement, coarse chromatic, and prominent nucleoli. Intracytoplasmic vacuoles containing neutrophils are noted (conventional preparation, Papanicolaou, ×400)

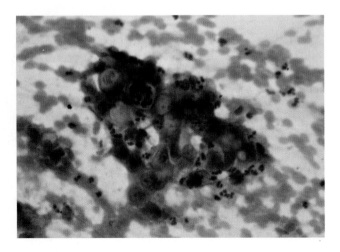

cells, and presence of abnormal endometrial cells. However, the first two features are too non-specific to be helpful.

Spontaneously shed benign appearing endometrial cells are often seen as part of the normal physiologic process during menses and the first part of the proliferative phase; they can be seen up to 10–12 days of the last menstrual period (LMP). Abnormal shedding of benign-appearing endometrial cells can be caused by a wide variety of conditions, including endometrial hyperplasias and carcinomas. Because of frequently missing clinical information such as the LMP, menopausal status, and hormonal therapy, TBS recommends the reporting of the exfoliated endometrial cells in women 40 years or older. Table 6.1 compares the terminologies used for reporting normal and abnormal endometrial cells in CV cytology.

The cytology of endometrial hyperplasias usually consists of one of the following scenarios:

**Table 6.3** Differential diagnosis of endocervical and endometrial adenocarcinoma

| Endocervical adenocarcinoma | Endometrial adenocarcinoma |
|---|---|
| 2-D honey comb sheets | Crowded 3-D clusters |
| Larger cells | Smaller cells |
| More variable | More uniform |
| Multinucleation: common | Multinucleation: rare |
| Fine, pale chromatin | Coarse, dark chromatin |
| Abundant cytoplasm | Scant cytoplasm |
| Well preserved | Degenerated |

the finding of cytologically normal endometrial cells out of phase in women of reproductive age, the finding of cytologically normal endometrial cells in postmenopausal women, and atypical endometrial cells. The cytology of endometrial adenocarcinomas varies with the degree of differentiation, ranging from abnormal shedding of cytologically normal endometrial cells for well differentiated tumors, to atypical endometrial cells, and to frank adenocarcinoma for poorly differentiated tumors. It is important to remember that the finding of cytologically benign endometrial cells in both pre- and postmenopausal women may be associated with a wide variety of conditions other than endometrial hyperplasias and adenocarcinomas.

Recently, some authors have advocated the use of direct endometrial sampling over exfoliative cytology for the detection of endometrial hyperplasias and adenocarcinomas. The advantages of direct sampling include high cellularity, more representative samples, and better preservation (Figs. 6.30 and 6.31). A high degree of sensitivity has been reported for diagnosing endometrial carcinoma. However, non-diagnostic samples can occur if the sampling devices cannot reach the uterine cavity because of a stenotic cervix. In addition, the use of direct endometrial sampling to diagnose endometrial hyperplasias has been quite disappointing.

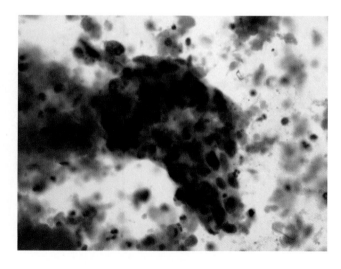

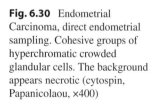

**Fig. 6.30** Endometrial Carcinoma, direct endometrial sampling. Cohesive groups of hyperchromatic crowded glandular cells. The background appears necrotic (cytospin, Papanicolaou, ×400)

**Fig. 6.31** Endometrial Carcinoma, direct endometrial sampling. Complex glandular structures composed of highly atypical glandular cells (cell block, H.E. ×100)

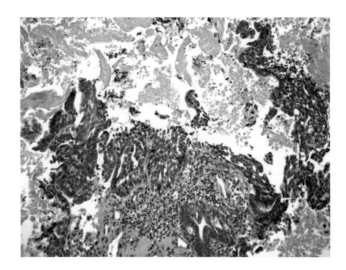

## 6.5.4 Hyperchromatic Crowded Groups

Hyperchromatic crowded groups (HCG) refer to the presence of irregular three-dimensional aggregates, which often appear darkly stained at low magnification. HCGs can pose considerable challenges to cytologists because they can be associated with both benign and neoplastic conditions (Table 6.4). Loss of nuclear polarity, haphazard cellular arrangement, coarse chromatin, irregular nuclear contours, and mitotic figures favor a neoplastic or preneoplastic process.

## Suggested Reading

Clement PB, Young RH. Endometrioid carcinoma of the uterine corpus. A review of its pathology with emphasis on recent advances and problematic aspects. Advances in Anatomic Pathology 2002, 9: 145–184.

Clement PB, Young RH. Non-endometrioid carcinomas of the uterine corpus: a review of their pathology with emphasis on recent advances and problematic aspects. Advances in Anatomic Pathology 2004, 11:117–142.

Diane S, Nayar R, Davey DD, Wilbur DC. The Bethesda System for Reporting Cervical Cytology: Definitions, Criteria, and Explanatory Notes. 2nd Edn. Springer, Berlin. 2004.

Demay RM. Hyperchromatic crowded groups: pitfalls in pap smear diagnosis. American Journal of Clinical Pathology 2000, 114 Suppl:S36–43.

Kurman R. Blaustein's Pathology of the Female Genital Tract. 5th Edn. Springer, Berlin. 2002.

Milojkovic M, et al. Assessment of reliability endometrial brush cytology in detection etiology of late postmenopausal bleedings. Archives of Gynecology and Obstetrics 2004, 269:259–262.

**Table 6.4** Differential diagnosis of hyperchromatic crowded groups

| Benign conditions |
| --- |
| Endocervical cells, particularly with liquid based preparation |
| Exfoliated endometrial cells |
| Lower uterine segment |
| Atrophy |
| Tubal metaplasia |
| Clusters of inflammatory cells |
| Neoplastic/preneoplastic |
| HSIL |
| AIS |
| Squamous-cell carcinoma |
| Adenocarcinoma |

# Chapter 7
# Nonepithelial Tumors of Uterine Corpus

**Keywords** Uterus • Nonepithelial • Sarcoma • Stromal tumors

## 7.1 General Classification of Nonepithelial Tumors of Uterine Corpus

Uterine mesenchymal tumors are generally divided into endometrial stromal tumors, smooth muscle tumors, mixed epithelial and stromal tumors, perivascular epithelioid-cell tumors and other mesenchymal tumors of both homologous and heterologous tissue types (Table 7.1).

## 7.2 Endometrial Stromal Tumors

Endometrial stromal tumors have proliferating cells with endometrial stromal differentiation at cytological and/or immunohistochemical levels. While high-grade endometrial stromal sarcoma is obviously malignant histologically, a separation of a low-grade endometrial stromal sarcoma from a benign endometrial stromal nodule is primarily determined by the presence invasive tumor border.

*Endometrial stromal nodule (ESN)* is a lesion of reproductive or postmenopausal women with a mean age of 47 years. Vaginal bleeding is the most common symptom. ESN is usually a single lesion that has a fleshy, tan to yellow cut surface and is sharply demarcated from surrounding endomyometrium (Fig. 7.1a). Histologically, the tumor is cellular and consists of benign looking endometrial stromal cells similar to those found in proliferative endometrium. The tumor cells are uniform and small with minimal cytological atypia (Fig. 7.1b). The nuclei are round to oval with fine chromatin and inconspicuous nucleoli. Mitosis is usually present, but less than 3 per 10 HPF. An even distribution of small vessels resembling spiral arterioles in normal endometrium is characteristic (Fig. 7.1b). Areas of tumor cells may appear spindlier to resemble fibroblasts or myofibroblasts and may be associated with marked collagen deposition as hyalinized plaques (Fig. 7.1c). Some tumors may have significant myxoid changes. Sex-cord differentiation, epithelioid tumor cells and atypical endometrial glands may also be seen. Histological examination of the entire tumor border is essential; implying a hysterectomy may be necessary when a diagnosis of ESN is considered in a biopsy or curettage. Focal finger-like protrusion of less than 3 mm is compatible with a diagnosis of ESN. An ESN with less than 9 mm border protrusion has been diagnosed as endometrial stromal tumor with limited infiltration, but the behavior of such lesions is uncertain. Immunohistochemically, the tumor cells express CD10, vimentin, and smooth muscle actin, ER, PR, and WT-1. Caldesmon is negative.

*Low grade endometrial stromal sarcoma* represents 15% of uterine sarcomas and two-third

**Table 7.1** Classifications of uterine non-epithelial tumors

| Major heading | Subheading | Subtype or variant | Subtype or variant | Subtype or variant | Subtype or variant |
|---|---|---|---|---|---|
| Endometrial stromal tumor | | Endometrial stromal nodule | Low-grade endometrial stromal tumor | High-grade endometrial stromal sarcoma | |
| Mixed endometrial stromal and smooth muscle tumor | | | | | |
| Mixed epithelial and stromal tumors | Adenomyoma | Atypical polypoid adenomyoma | | | |
| | Mullerian adenosarcoma | | | | |
| | Malignant mullerian mixed tumor | | | | |
| Smooth muscle tumor | Leiomyoma | Cellular leiomyoma | Mitotically active leiomyoma | Symplastic leiomyoma | Myxoid leiomyoma |
| | Leiomyosarcoma, conventional | | | | |
| | Smooth muscle tumor of uncertain malignant potential | | | | |
| | Epithelioid smooth muscle tumor | Plexiform tumorlet | Epithelioid leiomyoma | Epithelioid leiomyosarcoma | |
| | Myxoid smooth muscle tumor | | Myxoid leiomyoma | Myxoid leiomyosarcoma | |
| | Mature smooth muscle tumor with unusual presentation | Diffuse peritoneal leiomyomatosis | Dissecting leiomyoma | Intravascular leiomyomatosis | Metastasizing or parasitic leiomyoma |
| | | | Lymphangioleiomyomatosis | | |
| Perivascular epithelioid cell tumor | Conventional | Angiomyolipoma | | | |
| Other mesenchymal tumors | Homologous sarcoma | Angiosarcoma | Fibrosarcoma | Neurogenic sarcoma | |
| | Heterologous sarcoma | Rhabdomyosarcoma | Alveolar soft part sarcoma | Rhabdoid tumor | Epithelioid sarcoma |
| | Uterine tumor resembling ovarian sex-cord tumor | | | | |
| | Inflammatory myofibroblastic tumor | | | | |

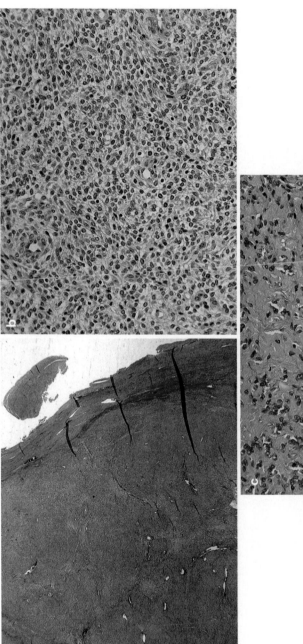

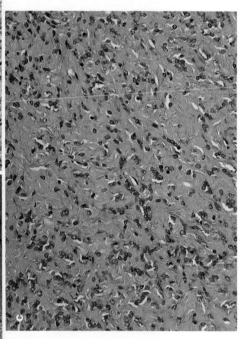

**Fig. 7.1** Endometrial stromal nodule (low power view, **a**, H.E. ×20). Note the sharp tumor border with the adjacent myometrium, characteristic tumor cells similar to those of the proliferative endometrium and the presence of evenly distributed arteriols (**b**, H.E. ×200) and hyalinized collagen deposition (**c**, H.E. ×200)

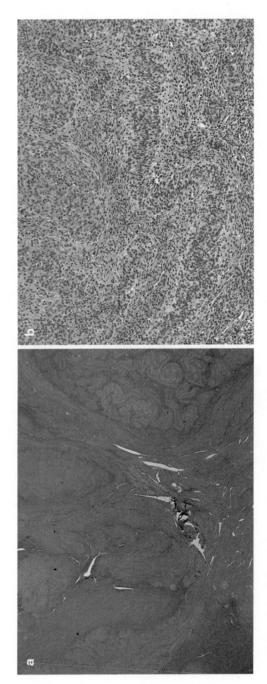

**Fig. 7.2** Low grade endometrial stromal sarcoma. Note the infiltrative tumor border with tongue-like tumor islands involving myometrium and lymphatics (**a**, H.E. ×20), and the sex cord differentiation in some tumors (**b**, H.E. ×100)

**Fig. 7.3** Endometrial stromal tumor with smooth muscle differentiation (stromomyoma) (H.E. ×40)

are seen in women less than 50 years of age. Vaginal bleeding and/or pelvic pain are common symptoms. The lesion may be polypoid or infiltrative myometrial mass with even grossly lymphovascular invasive by forming finger-like plugs within vasculatures that may extend into the parametrium. Microscopically, it essentially shares all the histological, immunohistochemical, and cytological features of ESN, except the presence of infiltrative border and tongue-like tumor growth involving adjacent myometrium and lymphovascular spaces (Fig. 7.2a), and hence the term "endolymphatic adenomyosis" in old literatures. Sex-cord differentiation is seen in about one-fifth of the cases (Fig. 7.2b).

*Endometrial stromal tumor with smooth muscle differentiation (stromomyoma)* requires the presence of at least 30% smooth muscle component for the diagnosis (Fig. 7.3). The smooth muscle component can be typical leiomyomatous or cellular proliferation of cells that needs immunohistochemical confirmation (desmin, caldesmon, and CD10). The presence of gapping vasculature is a helpful hint for the smooth muscle differentiation. Notably, it is the endometrial stromal component that dictates the biological behavior of the tumor. Similar to a conventional ESN, thorough assessment of the tumor border is essential.

*High-grade endometrial stromal sarcoma* is a diagnosis by exclusion, and some authors require

the presence of concurrent typical low-grade endometrial stromal sarcoma for such a diagnosis. Histologically, the tumor resembles a high-grade spindle-cell sarcoma with destructive growth pattern, necrosis, and high mitotic count (>10/10 HPF, Fig. 7.4a–c). Immunostaining is helpful to rule out leiomyosarcomas and rhabdomyosarcoma, but CD10 has not been found diagnostically useful.

## 7.3  Mullerian Mixed Epithelial and Stromal Tumors

*Typical adenomyoma* is a polypoid submucosal leiomyoma involved by endometriosis. The lesion consists of nodular smooth muscle proliferation interrupted by scattered benign proliferative type endometrial glands, some of which are surrounded by thin mantles of endometrial stroma.

*Atypical polypoid adenomyoma (APA)* is usually seen in premenopausal women with vaginal bleeding. The lesion frequently involves lower uterine segment or even cervix. Grossly resembling an endometrial polyp, APA consists of irregular hyperplastic endometrial glands embedded in a smooth muscle-rich stroma (Fig. 7.5a). The glandular epithelium focally shows mild to moderate cytological atypia including nuclear enlargement, hyperchromasia, loss of polarity,

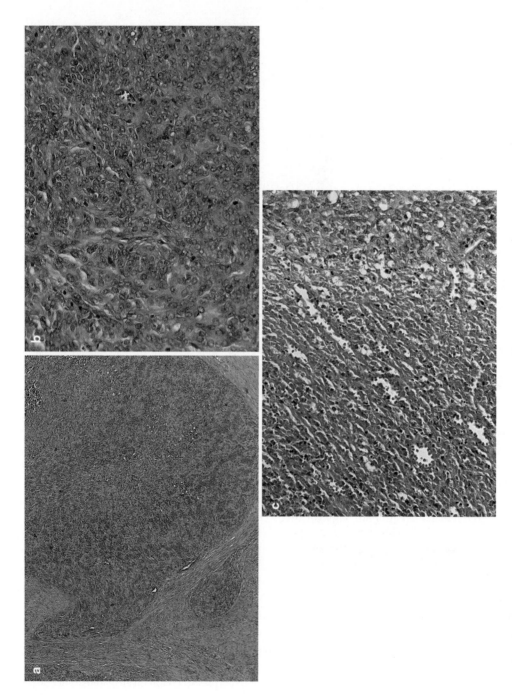

**Fig. 7.4** High grade endometrial stromal sarcoma. Note the high-grade spindle-cell proliferation with destructive growth pattern (**a**, H.E. ×40), cytological atypia, high mitotic count (**b**, H.E. ×200), and necrosis (**c**, H.E. ×200)

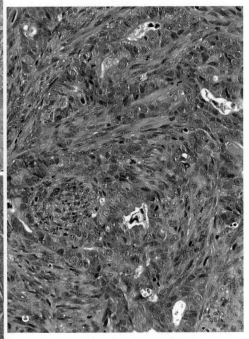

**Fig. 7.5** Atypical adenomyoma. Note the presence of hyperplastic endometrial glands embedded in a smooth muscle-rich stroma (**a**, H.E. ×40), and atypical endometrial glands with squamous metaplasia (**b**, H.E. ×200). Marked histological and cytological atypia in atypical polypoid adenomyoma of low malignant potential (**c**, H.E. ×200)

and cytoplasmic eosinophilia. Squamous differentiation is present in almost every case in the forms of immature squamous metaplasia to well developed squamous morules (Fig. 7.5b). They may be associated with focal keratinization and necrosis. The smooth muscles exist as boundless or fascicles and are cytologically benign. Occasional mitosis can be seen (2/10 HPF). APA with significant histological and cytological atypia has been diagnosed as atypical polypoid adenomyoma of low malignant potential (APA-LM, Fig. 7.5c). Well-differentiated invasive endometrioid carcinoma may coexist with or arise from an APA. APA, particularly APA-LM, recurs if not completely removed in about one-third to two-thirds of the cases. Hysterectomy is generally recommended, although conservative therapy is possible with polypectomy or curettage to preserve fertility as long as a close follow-up is in place.

*Mullerian adenosarcoma* is typically seen in a postmenopausal patient with vaginal bleeding and a polypoid endometrial mass. The tumor may fill up the entire endometrial cavity and protrude into the cervical os in half of the cases. Histologically, these are biphasic tumors with cystic glandular and sarcomatous components, generally in a broad based polypoid configuration with secondary branching, resembling phylloides tumor of the breast (Fig. 7.6a). The glandular epithelium is mostly proliferative endometrial type but tubal, endocervical, and metaplastic endometrial epithelium can also be seen. Although the glandular epithelium may show some atypicality, frank carcinomatous changes are not compatible with a diagnosis of adenosarcoma. The sarcomatous component is generally low-grade and consists of endometrial type stromal cells, but fibrosarcoma or even leiomyosarcomatous cells can be seen in some cases. The sarcomatous cells are characteristically condensing around or cuffing the cystically dilated glands (Fig. 7.6b). However, areas of the tumor may have deceptively benign hypocellular stromal component with marked hyalinization. Sex-cord differentiation and heterologous elements including cartilage, adipose, and rhabdomyoblasts are present in 20% of the cases.

The sarcomatous cells are usually positive for CD10, WT-1, ER, and PR. Diagnosis of adenosarcoma can be difficult. Recurrent misdiagnosis as endometrial or endocervical polyp occurs in some cases due to the deceptively benign appearance of the tumor in small biopsy or curettage specimens. The differential diagnosis should also include adenofibroma, a rare benign counterpart of adenosarcoma. High index of suspicion usually leads to a closer microscopic inspection of the specimen. The presence of two or more mitoses/10 HPF in stromal cells, periglandular cuffing by cellular stroma, and stromal cell atypicality should prompt a diagnosis of adenosarcoma. The tumor is limited to the uterus in almost every case at presentation. The presence of extrauterine tumor signifies the possibility of sarcomatous transformation/overgrowth.

*Malignant mullerian mixed tumor (MMMT) or carcinosarcoma* occurs almost exclusively in postmenopausal women, with vaginal bleeding and frequently high stage at presentation. The tumor represents less than 5% of uterine cancers and is now considered a variant of endometrial carcinoma undergoing malignant mesenchymal transdifferentiation. The tumor is typically a polypoid intrauterine mass with fleshy cut surface and extensive hemorrhage and necrosis. MMMT consists of intimately admixed carcinomatous and sarcomatous components in various proportions (Fig. 7.7a). The carcinomatous element is usually serous or endometrioid carcinoma. Clear cell, mucinous or undifferentiated carcinoma can also be seen. The sarcomatous element is generally high-grade sarcoma of either homologous (high grade endometrial stromal sarcoma, Fig. 7.7b) or heterologous (rhabdomyosarcoma, chondrosarcoma, osterosarcoma, and liposarcoma) nature (Fig. 7.7c, d). Immunohistochemistry can be helpful in identifying rare heterologous sarcomatous cells, particularly with rhabdomyosarcomatous differentiation. Pure carcinomatous lesions may be present adjacent to MMMT and sarcomatous component may be very focal, resulting in a diagnostic discrepancy between hysterectomy and endometrial curettage in some cases. Endometrioid carcinoma with spindle cell component should be

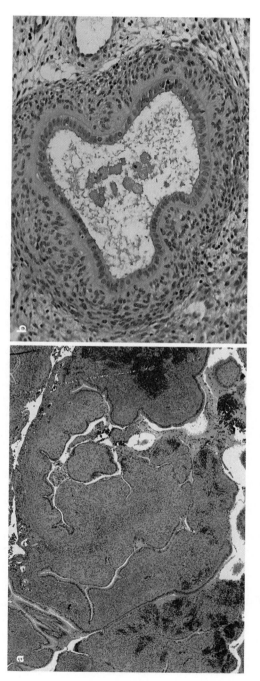

**Fig. 7.6** Adenosarcoma. Note the broad based polypoid configuration with secondary branching (**a**, H.E. ×40) and cellular stromal cuffing of the glands (**b**, H.E. ×200)

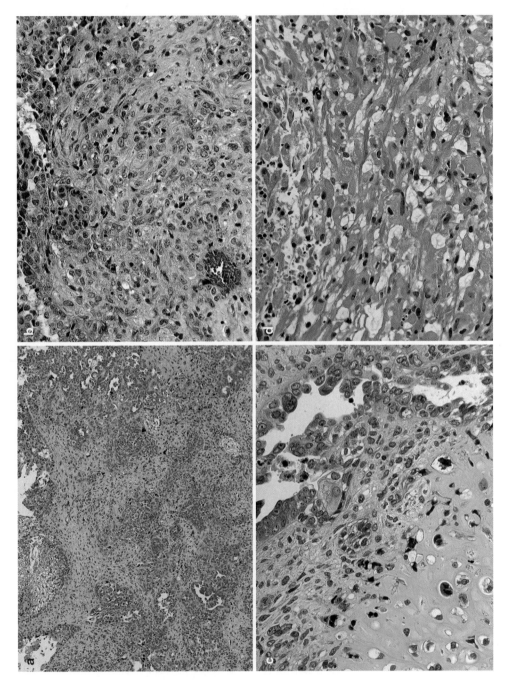

**Fig. 7.7** Malignant mixed mullerian tumor (MMT). The tumor consists of both carcinomatous and sarcomatous components (**a**, H.E. ×40). The sarcomatous element is generally high-grade sarcoma of either homologous (high grade endometrial stromal sarcoma, **b**, H.E. ×200) or heterologous nature, chondrosarcoma (**c**, H.E. ×200), and rhabdomyosarcoma (**d**, H.E. ×200) in this case

separated from MMMT by its low nuclear grade, gradual transition between typical endometrioid carcinoma glands to the spindle areas, absence of heterologous element and absence of rhabdomyomatous differentiation. MMMTs with unusual carcinomatous components such as squamous-cell carcinoma or adenoid basal-cell carcinoma are generally cervical primaries. MMMT is one of the most aggressive uterine malignancies with a 5-year survival of only 5–40% and a median survival of less than 2 years. Recurrent or metastatic tumor can be pure carcinomatous (the most common), pure sarcomatous, or both components of the primary MMMT.

## 7.4 Smooth Muscle Tumors

Smooth muscle tumors (Table 7.1) of the uterus are generally divided into benign leiomyomas, malignant leiomyosarcomas, and subsets of tumors with low malignant potential (smooth muscle tumor of uncertain malignant potential), unusual clinical behaviors (benign metastasizing leiomyoma, diffuse peritoneal leiomyomatosis, and peritoneal/parasitic leiomyoma), and those with unique growth patterns (intravenous leiomyomatosis, uterine leiomyomatosis, and dissecting leiomyomas/cotyledonoid leiomyoma).

*Leiomyoma* is the most common tumor of the uterus in general and is found in about two-third of hysterectomy specimens. Clinical symptoms (vaginal bleeding, pelvic pain, or pressure related disorders) are results of the tumor size, number and location. Leiomyomas are multiple in two-thirds of the cases and subdivided into submucosal, mural, and subserosal tumors. They are well circumscribed without capsule, and rubbery firm. Cut surfaces are often bulging, white in color, and solid. However, many degenerative leiomyomas have various colors (red, brown, yellow, and hemorrhagic) and texture (edematous, fleshy to obviously necrotic). Conventional leiomyomas consist of fascicles or bundles of elongated spindle cells with eosinophilic cytoplasm and a centrally located cigar shaped nucleus (Fig. 7.8). Interstitial collagen may be present and in a long-standing leiomyoma, there may be significant amount of hyalinized collagen. Vasculatures are typically rich within the tumor of various calibers and types (muscle-rich arteries, arteriols, and veins). Large gapping vasculatures are typical findings.

Secondary histological changes are common in a leiomyoma. Infarction type necrosis typically displays zonal configurations, in which necrotic smooth muscle cells are surrounded by rims of granulation to fibrous tissue with varying degrees of hyalinization (Fig. 7.9). Coagulative or tumor-cell necrosis should not present in a leiomyoma (see leiomyosarcomas). Infarction type necrosis combined with intratumoral hemorrhage (red degeneration) is commonly seen in

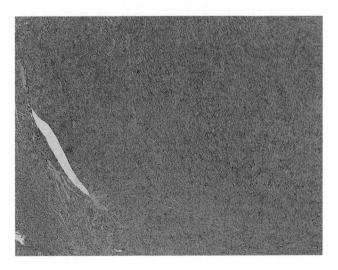

**Fig. 7.8** Leiomyoma. Conventional leiomyomas consists of fascicles or bundles of elongated spindle cells with eosinophilic cytoplasm and a centrally located cigar shaped nucleus (H.E. ×40)

**Fig. 7.9** Leiomyoma with
hyalinizing necrosis. Note the zonal
configurations where necrotic
smooth muscle cells are surrounded
by rims of granulation to fibrous
tissue with varying degrees of
hyalinization (H.E. ×40)

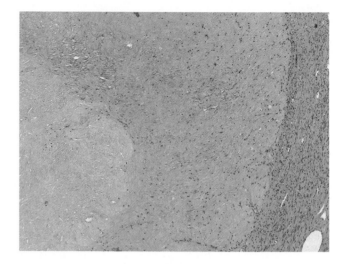

**Fig. 7.10** Cellular leiomyoma
(H.E. ×40)

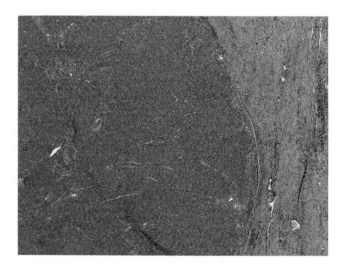

patients receiving hormonal treatment or with concurrent pregnancy. In such condition, histologically, the leiomyoma may have active smooth muscle proliferation with increased mitotic activity around the infarction type necrosis. Infarction type necrosis can also been seen secondary to uterine artery embolization by polyvinyl alcohol for treatment of symptomatic leiomyomas. Identification of the foreign materials along with giant cell reaction points to a correct diagnosis.

Leiomyomas with unusual histological patterns are common diagnostic problems. Cellular leiomyoma has a hypercellularity that is significantly higher than that of adjacent myometrium.

But the tumor should not have cytological atypia, necrosis, or more than 4 mitoses per 10 HPF (Fig. 7.10). Highly cellular leiomyoma has even higher cellularity with short spindle cells, frequently resembling an endometrial stromal tumor. The presence of vague fascicular growth pattern, clefting spaces, and thickened arteries favor a leiomyoma over an endometrial stromal tumor. Desmin and caldesmon positivity confirms a smooth-muscle tumor. Positive CD10 immunostain is seen in near half of the cases. Leiomyoma with bizarre nuclei or symplastic leiomyoma is a conventional leiomyoma with scattered foci of large atypical smooth-muscle cells that have abundant eosinophilic cytoplasm, bizarre nuclear

**Fig. 7.11** Leiomyoma with bizarre nuclei or symplastic leiomyoma. Note the hyperchromatic and degenerative nuclei, often with intranuclear inclusions (H.E. ×200)

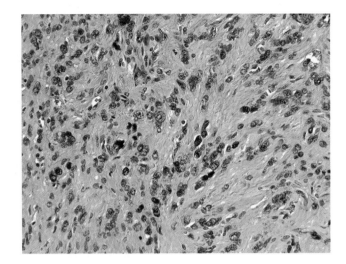

**Fig. 7.12** Plexiform tumorlet. Note the plexiform configuration of nests and cords of polygonal epithelioid cells (H.E. ×40)

shapes, and multinucleation (Fig. 7.11). The chromatin of the bizarre cells is hyperchromatic and degenerative in nature, often with intranuclear inclusions. Further degeneration may lead to additional chromatin condensation and fragmentation, simulating atypical mitotic figures. However, bona fide mitoses are less than 10 per 10 HPF. Negative P16, low mib-1, and euploidy may be helpful for its separation from a leiomyosarcoma. Mitotically active leiomyoma is an otherwise conventional leiomyoma, but with 4–20 mitosis per 10 HPF. The tumor may be associated with high hormonal status (secretory phase, pregnancy, or taking exogenous hormone). "Leiomyoma with increased mitotic index but experience limited" has been proposed for similar tumors with more than 20 mitoses per 10 HPF. Myxoid leiomyoma needs to be separated from a myxoid leiomyosarcoma by its well-circumscribed border, absence of nuclear atypia, no coagulative tumor necrosis and absence of mitotic activity. Epithelioid leiomyoma consists of eosinophilic polygonal smooth-muscle cells that can involve focally or diffusely a conventional leiomyoma. Its microscopic variant, plexiform tumorlet, is often an incidental microscopic finding within the myometrium and consists of nests and cords of polygonal epithelioid cells (Fig. 7.12). Lipoleiomyoma has an integral component of mature adipose tissue (Fig. 7.13).

**Fig. 7.13** Lipoleiomyoma. Note the integral mixture of smooth muscle and mature fat cells in the tumor (H.E. ×40)

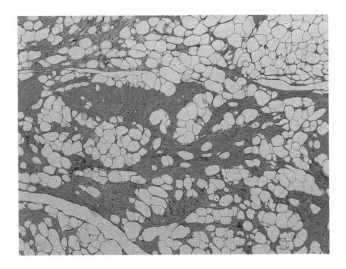

**Fig. 7.14** Intravenous leiomyomatosis. Note the smooth muscle proliferation tracking and plugging numerous vasculatures, and endothelial covered tumor plugs show tissue molding, clefting and hyalinization (H.E. ×40)

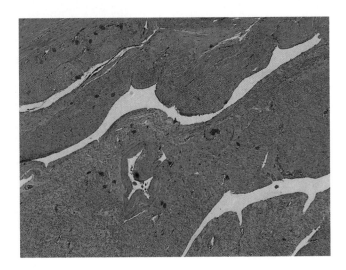

Focal or diffuse stromal edema in otherwise conventional leiomyoma can be named hydropic leiomyoma.

*Intravenous leiomyomatosis* is a well-differentiated smooth muscle tumor that has an unusual intravenous growth pattern inside and outside of the uterus. The tumor is frequently an irregular myometrial mass with tumor plugs within vasculatures that may extend into parametrial or pelvic veins in 30% of the cases, and occasionally further into the vena cava and right ventricle. Microscopically, the serpentine smooth muscle bundles proliferate, tracking and plugging numerous vasculatures, at the tumor periphery and beyond. Endothelial covered tumor plugs show tissue molding, clefting, hyalinization, and rich vasculatures (Fig. 7.14).

*Diffuse peritoneal leiomyomatosis* is rare smooth muscle proliferation characterized by the presence of several to multiple peritoneal nodules of leiomyomas of less than 1 cm in size. The condition is typically found young patients with concurrent or recent pregnancy during cesarean section or tubal ligation. The proliferating smooth muscle cells may show occasional mitosis, but significant cytological atypia and

**Fig. 7.15**  Metastasizing
leiomyoma involving lung
(H.E. ×40)

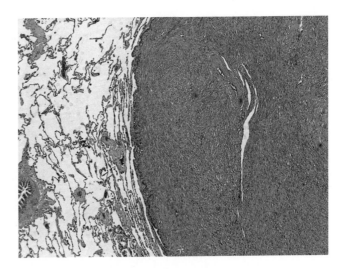

tumor-cell necrosis are absent. The condition is self-limiting, even without complete removal of all tumor nodules at the surgery.

*Benign metastasizing leiomyoma* is a conventional uterine leiomyoma with concurrent extra-uterine tumors of similar histology, frequently involving lung (Fig. 7.15) and rarely retroperitoneal and mediastinal lymph nodes, bone and soft tissue. The diagnosis requires a thorough sampling and histological examination to exclude a leiomyosarcoma of the uterus.

*Dissecting leiomyoma* has a dissecting growth pattern with bundles of proliferating smooth-muscle cells protruding and splitting the uterine myometrium. In extremely rare cases, the dissecting muscle bundles may extend outside of the uterus into the broad ligament, forming a large mushroom-like mass (cotyledonoid variant). The condition is benign.

*Leiomyosarcomas* of the uterus are highly malignant sarcomas usually found in an adult woman. Generally a solitary large mass (average of 10 cm), most leiomyosarcomas are de novo, despite of their frequent coexistence with multiple leiomyomas. The tumor has an infiltrative border and a fleshy, bulging cut surface that usually has necrosis and hemorrhage. Histologically, most leiomyosarcomas are overtly malignant tumors that are not diagnostically difficult. The majority of leiomyosarcomas demonstrate marked cellularity, moderate to severe cytological atypia

(appreciable at low to medium power), mitosis of 10 or more per 10 HPF and coagulative tumor-cell necrosis (Fig. 7.16a, b). The presence of coagulative tumor-cell necrosis essentially establishes a diagnosis of leiomyosarcoma until proven otherwise. In contrast to the infarction type necrosis in a benign leiomyoma, coagulative tumor necrosis has an irregular geographic pattern with abrupt transition between viable and necrotic ghost tumor cells. Characteristically, necrotic areas are punctuated by discernable vasculatures, and some of the vessels may be cuffed by viable tumor cells (Fig. 7.17). In the absence of coagulative tumor necrosis, moderate to severe cytological atypia combined with 10 or more mitotic count per 10 HPF also establishes the diagnosis of leiomyosarcoma (Fig. 7.18). Poorly differentiated leiomyosarcomas may require smooth muscle markers to establish the muscle nature. High levels of P16 and Mib-1 are features of leiomyosarcoma. p53 positivity can also be seen in a leiomyosarcoma, but not leiomyoma and its variants.

*Epithelioid leiomyosarcomas* have, similar to its benign counterpart, polygonal tumor cells with abundant eosinophilic cytoplasm. Obvious cytological atypia, mitotic count of 4 or more per 10 HPF and the presence of coagulative tumor-cell necrosis establish a diagnosis of malignancy (Fig. 7.19a, b). Immunohistochemistry study of smooth muscle marker and epithelial markers can be misleading.

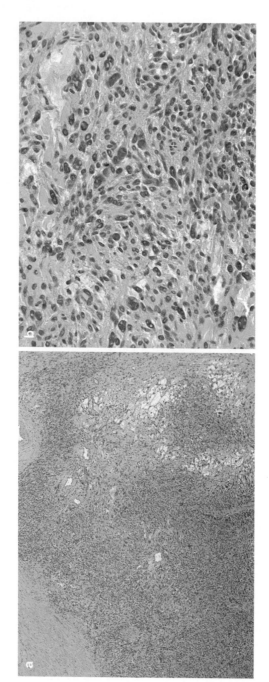

**Fig. 7.16** (**a**, **b**) Leiomyosarcomas. Note the marked cellularity, moderate to severe cytological atypia (appreciable at low to medium power, mitosis of 10 to more per 10 HPF and coagulative tumor-cell necrosis) (**a**, H.E. ×40; **b**, H.E. ×200)

**Fig. 7.17** Coagulative tumor necrosis. Note irregular geographic pattern with abrupt transition between viable and necrotic ghost tumor cells (H.E. ×200)

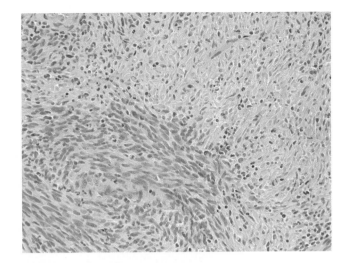

**Fig. 7.18** Leiomyosarcoma with moderate to severe cytological atypia combined with 10 or more mitotic count per 10 HPF

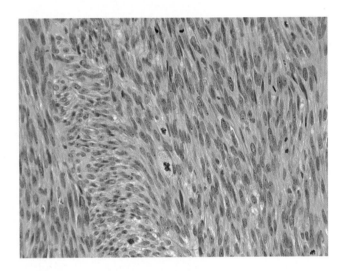

*Myxoid leiomyosarcomas* are edematous and hypocellular tumors with an infiltrative border. They have relatively small spindle cells with hyperchromatic nuclei and scant cytoplasm. The presence of tumor cells with smooth muscle differentiation can usually be found in nonmyxoid area. The presence of tumor-cell necrosis, a mitotic index of 2 or more per 10 HPF, and nuclear atypia are features of malignancy (Fig. 7.20).

Smooth muscle tumors with borderline features between leiomyoma and leiomyosarcomas are diagnosed under the umbrella "*smooth muscle tumors of uncertain malignancy potential or STUMP*" due to their unpredictable clinical behaviors. Frequent scenarios include a smooth muscle tumor with diffuse moderate cytological atypia and a mitotic count of less than 10 per 10 HPF (Fig. 7.21a); an otherwise conventional leiomyoma with necrosis of uncertain type (Fig. 7.21b); and an otherwise conventional leiomyoma or cellular leiomyoma with mitotic counts of more than 20 per 10 HPF (Fig. 7.21c).

## 7.5 Other Mesenchymal Tumors

Various soft tissue tumors may rarely occur in uterus including vascular tumors, fibrohistiocytic tumors, neurogenic tumors and rhabdomyosarcoma,

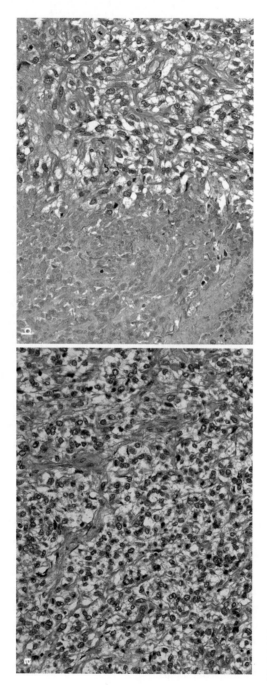

**Fig. 7.19** Epithelioid leiomyosarcoma. Note the polygonal tumor cells with abundant eosinophilic cytoplasm (**a**, H.E. ×200) and the presence of coagulative tumor-cell necrosis (**b**, H.E. ×200)

**Fig. 7.20** Myxoid leiomyosarcomas. Note the edematous and hypocellular proliferation of spindle cells with hyperchromatic nuclei and scant cytoplasm (H.E. ×40)

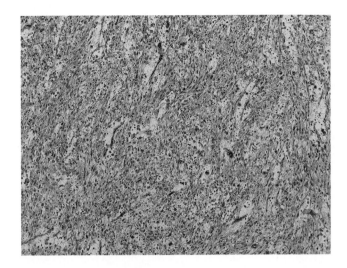

malignant rhabdoid tumor, epithelioid sarcoma, and alveolar soft part sarcoma. Uterine tumor resembling ovarian sex-cord tumor, inflammatory myofibroblastic tumor, and perivascular epithelioid tumors are ones that are relatively distinct and well characterized in uterus.

*Uterine tumor resembling ovarian sex-cord tumor (UTROSCT)* is an uncommon lesion of adulthood, typically presenting with vaginal bleeding. The tumor may be a well circumscribed myometrial lesion or a polypoid endometrial mass. Histologically, the tumor is characterized by the proliferation of epithelioid cells resembling ovarian sex-cord tumors, particularly granulosa cell or Sertolic cell tumors (Fig. 7.22a). The epithelioid tumor cells are generally small and round without significant cytological atypia or mitosis. They form anatomizing cords, small nests, tubules, or even retiform pattern (Fig. 7.22b). Areas resembling sex-cord differentiation may have larger tumor cells with abundant foamy cytoplasm, closely resembling luteinized cells. Varying amount of fibromyomatous stromal component can be found. The most common immunohistochemical profile of the tumor is the combined positivity of cytokeratin, EMA, vimentin, one or more smooth muscle markers (desmin, SMA, and caldesmon), one or more sex-core makers (calretinin, CD99, inhibin, Melan-A, WT-1, and CD10), and hormone markers (ER and PR). UTROSCT is a borderline to low-grade tumor with a recurrent rate of 15% after hysterectomy.

*Inflammatory myofibroblastic tumor (IMT)* involves endometrium as a polypoid lesion or myometrium as a mass lesion. It consists of fascicles or lobules of spindle myofibroblasts admixed with lymphoplasmacytes and extravasated red cells (Fig. 7.23). The diagnosis is confirmed by a positive ALK immunostain. Smooth muscle markers may be negative, so as ER. Molecular demonstration of ALK gene translocation by fluorescence in-situ hybridization can also be diagnostic.

*Perivascular epithelioid tumor (PECOMA)* may resemble a leiomyoma grossly and histologically. The tumor consists of spindle to epithelioid cells with clear to eosinophilic cytoplasm, arranged in sheets or fascicles. The tumor is generally highly vascularized. The tumor cells are by definition positive for melanocytic markers (HMB-45, Melan-A, or microphthalmia transcription factor) and smooth muscle cell markers (desmin). The tumor is benign in most cases, but a third are clinically malignant. Features of malignancy include more than 5 cm in size, infiltrative border, markedly atypicality, necrosis, and more than 1 mitosis per 50 HPF.

## 7.6  Cytology

Primary, nonepithelial malignant neoplasms of the uterine corpus are uncommon and may rarely be seen in gynecologic cytology. Only a few of these

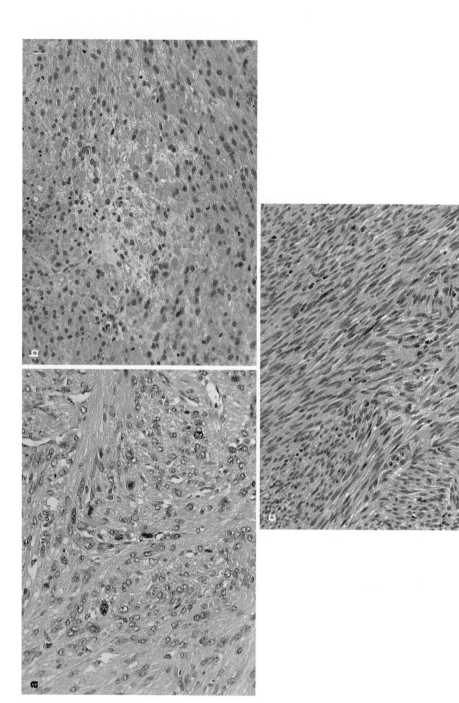

**Fig. 7.21** Smooth muscle tumors of uncertain malignancy potential or STUMP. Smooth muscle tumor with diffuse moderate cytological atypia and a mitotic count of less than 10 per 10 HPF (**a**, H.E. ×200); an otherwise conventional leiomyoma with necrosis of uncertain type (**b**, H.E. ×200); an otherwise conventional leiomyoma or cellular leiomyoma with mitotic counts of more than 20 per 10 HPF (**c**, H.E. ×200)

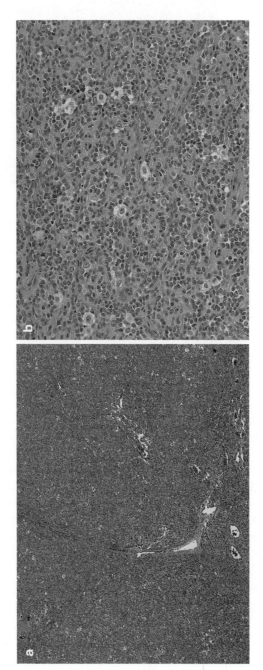

**Fig. 7.22** Uterine tumor resembling ovarian sex-cord tumor (UTROSCT). The tumor is characterized by the proliferation of epithelioid cells resembling ovarian sex-cord tumors, particularly granulosa cell or Sertolic cell tumors (**a** H.E. ×40). The epithelioid tumor cells are generally small and round without significant cytological atypia or mitosis. They form anatomizing cords, small nests, tubules or even retiform pattern (**b** H.E. ×200)

**Fig. 7.23** Inflammatory myofibroblastic tumor. Note the fascicles or lobules of spindle myofibrolasts admixed with lymphoplasmacytes (H.E. ×200)

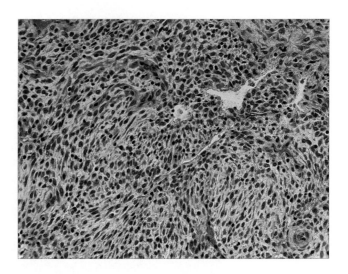

tumors may present characteristic features to allow a definitive diagnosis based on morphology alone. For the majority of these tumors, a definitive diagnosis is usually impossible because of limited sampling and morphologic overlap with other entities.

### 7.6.1 Sarcomas

Uterine sarcomas seldom exfoliated. In addition, their cytology varies depending on the histologic subtypes and the grade of the sarcomas. For example, the neoplastic cells of low grade endometrial stromal sarcomas resemble that of normal endometrial stromal cells with minimal cytologic atypia. On the contrary, marked cytologic atypia is usually observed with leiomyosarcoma, high grade endometrial stromal sarcomas, and malignant mixed mullerian tumors (MMMT). The latter may demonstrate a biphasic pattern of carcinoma and sarcoma.

### 7.6.2 Melanoma

The cytology is similar to those occurring in other parts of the body. The typical presentation

is isolated and loosely cohesive large epithelioId cells with abundant eosinophilic cytoplasm, and round to oval nuclei with prominent nucleoli. Occasionally, spindle-shaped neoplastic cells can be seen. The differential diagnosis includes poorly differentiated carcinoma, lymphoma, and sarcoma.

### 7.6.3 Lymphoma

Both Hodgkin's and non-Hodgkin's lymphomas have been described in gynecologic cytology; however, the latter are more frequent. Non-Hodgkin's lymphomas typically present with a monotonous population of lymphocytes. The differential diagnoses include follicular cervicitis, small-cell carcinoma, and poorly differentiated carcinoma.

### 7.6.4 Metastatic Tumors

Metastatic tumors to the uterine cervix also occur rarely. Knowledge of a prior malignancy and comparison with prior pathologic materials are helpful in arriving at the correct diagnosis.

## Suggested Reading

Clement PB. The pathology of uterine smooth muscle tumors and mixed endometrial stromal-smooth muscle tumors: a selective review with emphasis on recent advances. Int J Gynecol Pathol. 2000, 19:39–55.

Kempson R, Hendrickson MR. Smooth muscle, endometrial stromal, and mixed Mullerian tumors of the uterus. Mod Pathol. 2000, 13:328–342.

Kurman RJ. Blaustein's Pathology of the Female Genital Tract. 5th Edition. Springer, Berlin. 2002.

# Chapter 8
# Gestational Trophoblastic Disease

**Keywords** Trophoblastic disease • Hydatidiform mole • Choriocarcinoma

## 8.1 General Classification of Gestational Trophoblastic Disease

Gestational trophoblastic disease (GTD) encompasses a spectrum of proliferative disorders ranging from non-neoplastic hydatidiform moles to neoplastic conditions including the highly malignant gestational choriocarcinoma (CC). Two distinct tumors of the intermediate trophoblasts are very rare, but frequently pose diagnostic difficulties. In addition, two reactive conditions are also included in the classifications of GTDs (Table 8.1).

## 8.2 Hydatidiform Moles

Hydatidiform moles are non-neoplastic proliferations of the villous trophoblasts and characterized by enlarged hydropic villi along with trophoblastic hyperplasia. They are incompatible with fetal survival and genetically defined by their unique parental chromosome contributions. The two main subtypes are complete hydatidiform mole (CHM) and partial hydatidiform mole (PHM). Invasive hydatidiform mole is the one that invades myometrium. Persistent GTD is a clinical diagnosis, including invasive mole or metastatic mole that may develop following either CHM or PHM.

### 8.2.1 Complete Hydatidiform Mole

Patients with fully developed CHM present generally in the second trimester of pregnancy with vaginal bleeding, enlarged uterine size, markedly elevated serum human chorionic gonadotropin (hCG), hyperemesis, toxemia, and hyperthyroidism. Voluminous hydropic chorionic villi are typically gross findings. Markedly edematous villi with central cistern formation, diffuse circumferential trophoblastic hyperplasia involving both cytotrophoblasts and syncytiotrophoblasts, and cytological atypia are characteristic findings (Fig. 8.1). However, modern maternity care has drastically changed the clinical and histological presentations of complete mole due to early evacuation of molar tissue, typically during the first trimester. In these early complete mole, the chorionic villi are smaller and remarkably "cauliflower-like" or polypoid in configurations (Fig. 8.2). The villous stroma is characteristically hypercellular, composed of stellate fibroblasts embedded in a bluish myxoid matrix with prominent karyorrhexis. Trophoblastic hyperplasia is only focally present or may be entirely absent.

D. Chhieng and P. Hui (eds.), *Cytology and Surgical Pathology of Gynecologic Neoplasms*, Current Clinical Pathology, DOI 10.1007/978-1-60761-164-6_8, © Springer Science+Business Media, LLC 2011

**Table 8.1** Classification of gestational trophoblastic diseases

|  | Subtype | Subtype | Subtype |
| --- | --- | --- | --- |
| Hydatidiform mole | Complete | Partial | Invasive |
| Gestational choriocarcinoma |  |  |  |
| Placental site trophoblastic tumor (PSTT) |  |  |  |
| Epithelioid trophoblastic tumor (ETT) |  |  |  |
| Exaggerated placental site (EPS) reaction |  |  |  |
| Placental site nodule (PSN) | Atypical PSN |  |  |

Diagnostic separation of CHM, particularly very early complete mole, from hydropic non-molar gestations, early gestational sac, and PHM is often challenging. Demonstration of diploidy by DNA flow cytometry is the most frequently used method to distinguish CHM from triploid PHM. Hydropic abortuses and PHMs show strong nuclear p57 expression in cytotrophoblasts and villous stromal, whereas p57 staining is absent or very low in CHMs. Molecular genotyping is the most recently validated technique that can precisely diagnose and subtype molar pregnancies by demonstrating paternal-only genome in a

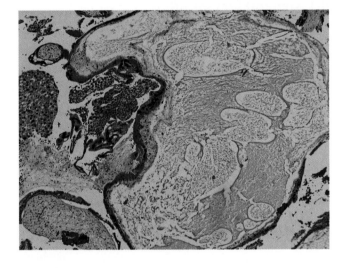

**Fig. 8.1** Well developed complete mole. Note the markedly edematous villi with central cistern formation, trophoblastic hyperplasia involving both cytotrophoblasts and syncytiotrophoblasts, and trophoblastic atypia (H.E. ×40)

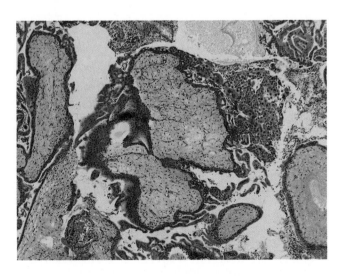

**Fig. 8.2** Very early complete mole shows polypoid chorionic villi with mild trophoblastic hyperplasia, and cellular myxoid villous stroma (H.E. ×40)

complete mole or triploid, diandric, and monogynic genome in a partial mole.

## 8.2.2 Partial Hydatidiform Mole

Majority of the patients present in the late first trimester or early second trimester with missed or incomplete abortion. The uterine size is usually small or appropriate for gestational age. Serum hCG is usually moderately elevated and a fetus may be seen by ultrasound. Microscopically, there are two populations of villi: large, hydropic, irregular villi in the background of small and fibrotic villi (Fig. 8.3). The larger villi show hydropic changes with central cistern formation, irregular/scalloped contour and trophoblastic inclusions. The trophoblastic hyperplasia is usually mild and focal, and lack significant nuclear atypia. Fetal blood vessels and nucleated red blood cells are commonly seen.

Gestations with chromosomal abnormalities (particularly trisomies 13, 15, 18, 21, and 22) may show villous enlargement, cavitation, surface scalloping, and trophoblastic inclusions, closely resembling PHM. Rarely, twin gestations with CHM and coexisting fetus can be mistaken for PHM as there are two populations of villi: molar villi from the CHM and normal villi from the normal twin. Placental mesenchymal dysplasia or "pseudo-partial mole" is characterized by stem villous and terminal villous hydrops, aneurysmal stem villous vessels, peripheral stem villous chorioangiomatoid change, and absence of trophoblastic hyperplasia. DNA ploidy analysis is useful in diagnosing a triploid gestation, but is unable to distinguish triploid, diandric, and monogynic PHMs from triploid digynic non-molar gestations. Molecular genotyping offers a highly accurate and reliable method to differentiate PHMs from non-molar triploid gestations.

## 8.2.3 Invasive Hydatidiform Mole

Complete and PHMs may progress into invasive or metastatic moles in approximately 15–20% and 0.5–4% of cases, respectively. Both invasive and metastatic hydatidiform moles present clinically as persistent GTD with constantly elevated serum hCG. The diagnosis therefore is often a clinical one, not requiring a pathologic confirmation. In rare cases where hysterectomy is performed, molar villi invading the myometrium without intervening decidua are diagnostic. Rarely, molar villi also invade intramyometrial vessels and may spread to vagina, vulva, and the broad ligament. Lung metastases can also develop.

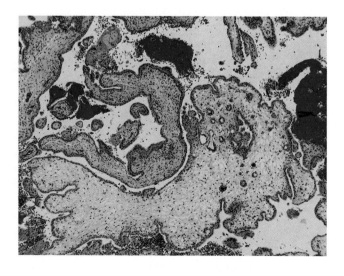

**Fig. 8.3** Well-developed partial molar demonstrates two populations (enlarged hydropic and normal sized fibrotic) of villi, surface scalloping and round to oval trophoblastic inclusions, minimal trophoblastic hyperplasia in the forms of syncytiotrophoblast knuckles or aggregates (H.E. ×40)

**Fig. 8.4** Gestational
choriocarcinoma consists
of destructive proliferation of
markedly atypical cytotrophoblasts
and syncytiotrophoblasts
in a bilamellar growth pattern
(H.E. ×40)

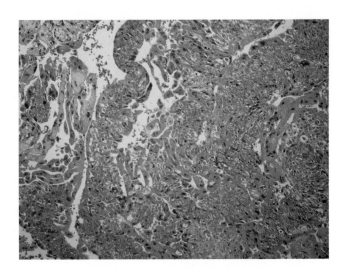

## 8.3 Gestational Choriocarcinoma

Choriocarcinoma is the most aggressive form of
gestational trophoblastic neoplasia with high pro-
pensity for hematogenous spread. It may develop
following hydatidiform mole, abortion, normal
gestation, or an ectopic pregnancy in 50, 25, 22.5,
and 2.5% of the cases, respectively. Grossly, choriocarcinoma is a highly hemorrhagic and often
necrotic mass lesion with a destructive border. On
microscopic examination, the tumor has a characteristic biphasic appearance (Fig. 8.4): central
sheets of cytotrophoblasts are surrounded by a rim
of syncytiotrophoblasts, but sometimes more haphazard arrangements of the two components may
be seen. Intermediate trophoblasts are also present
in variable proportions. There is marked nuclear
atypia, often with bizarre trophoblastic nuclei and
atypical mitotic figures. Vascular invasion is common. Chorionic villi are absent. Choriocarcinoma
must be distinguished from the previllous trophoblasts of a very early gestation, and the remnant
of hyperplastic trophoblasts of a complete mole
after most of the molar villi have been evacuated.

## 8.4 Placental Site Trophoblastic Tumor

Placental site trophoblastic tumor (PSTT) is a
neoplastic proliferation of extravillous (intermediate) trophoblasts at the implantation site.

It usually occurs during the reproductive years,
months to several years after an antecedent term
pregnancy, abortion, or a hydatidiform mole.
Patients usually present with irregular vaginal
bleeding or amenorrhea and asymmetric uterine enlargement. The tumor grossly appears as
a soft, tan-white, or yellow infiltrative mass
involving endomyometrium, occasionally with
foci of hemorrhage and necrosis. The tumor
sizes range from 0.7–10 cm. Microscopic
examination reveals atypical intermediate trophoblasts infiltrating the myometrium as single
cells, aggregates, or cords splitting apart individual smooth muscle fibers (Fig. 8.5). The
tumor cells are predominantly mononucleate,
but binucleate and multinucleate forms are
common. Moderate to severe nuclear atypia
and mitotic activity are usually present. High
mitotic activity (over 5 mitoses/10 HPF) has
been found to be associated with worse prognosis. Necrosis may focally be present. PSTTs
generally show diffuse immunostaining with
intermediate trophoblastic markers, i.e. hPL,
HLA-G, and Mel-CAM (CD146), whereas
expression of hCG and inhibin is only focal.
The presence of infiltrating margin, intimate
admixture of tumor cells with smooth muscle
fibers, diffuse hPL positivity, and negative p63
separate PSTT from epithelioid trophoblastic
tumor (ETT) (see below). Majority of PSTTs
are cured by hysterectomy. However, 10–15%
of the cases recur or develop metastases, most
commonly to the lung.

**Fig. 8.5** PSTT demonstrates an infiltrative proliferation of atypical implantation intermediate trophoblasts involving myometrium. The tumor cells are large mononuclear cells with abundant eosinophilic or clear cytoplasm and centrally located convoluted nuclei (H.E. ×200)

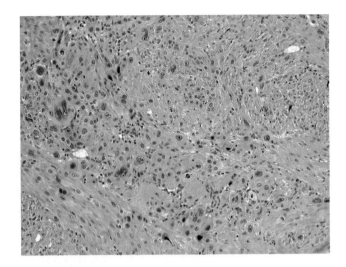

## 8.5 Epithelioid Trophoblastic Tumor

ETT is very rare trophoblastic tumor arising from the intermediate trophoblasts of the chorion laeve. The clinical features of ETT are very similar to those of PSTT: patients usually present during the reproductive years with abnormal vaginal bleeding and mild to moderate elevation of serum hCG. The tumor may develop 1–18 years (mean 6.2) after a full-term delivery, spontaneous abortion, or a molar pregnancy. ETT appears as a relatively well-defined tan to brown nodule involving endomyometrium or endocervix. Microscopically, the lesion is typically expansile and consists of solid nests and sheets of mononuclear intermediate trophoblastic cells. Central or irregular areas of tumor nests frequently contain eosinophilic, hyalinized material, and necrotic debris resembling keratin (Fig. 8.6a). The tumor cells are fairly uniform with mild to moderate nuclear atypia and relatively abundant eosinophilic or clear cytoplasm (Fig. 8.6b). The mitotic activity generally ranges from 1–10/10 HPF, but rarely may be as high as 48/10 HPF. The tumor cells may colonize the surface mucosa of the cervix, simulating cervical squamous intraepithelial neoplasia. Interestingly, decidualized benign stromal cells are frequently found around the tumor nests. Immunohistochemical stains for trophoblastic differentiation – hPL, Mel-CAM, inhibin, and hCG – show only focal positivity. HLA-G expression

may be focal or absent. However, P63 staining demonstrates a strong, diffuse, nuclear staining pattern. ETT is frequently misdiagnosed as invasive carcinoma due to its frequent endocervical location, epithelioid morphology, and presence of eosinophilic material mimicking keratin. Young patient's age, low level of hCG, absence of true keratin or cervical intraepithelial neoplasia, stromal decidual changes, and positivity of trophoblastic markers (inhibin, hPL, and hCG) are findings sufficiently separating an ETT from a carcinoma. Most ETTs behave in a benign fashion, but local recurrence and metastases occur in approximately 25% of cases. Similarly to PSTT, the primary treatment is hysterectomy and combined chemotherapy has been successful for metastatic disease.

## 8.6 Exaggerated Placental Site Reaction

Exaggerated placental site (EPS) reaction is likely a reactive process, usually seen with concurrent pregnancy or molar gestation, particularly complete mole. It shares many features of PSTT – including infiltrative growth pattern of proliferating intermediate trophoblasts, vascular invasion by trophoblasts, and presence of extracellular fibrinoid material (Fig. 8.7). It may be

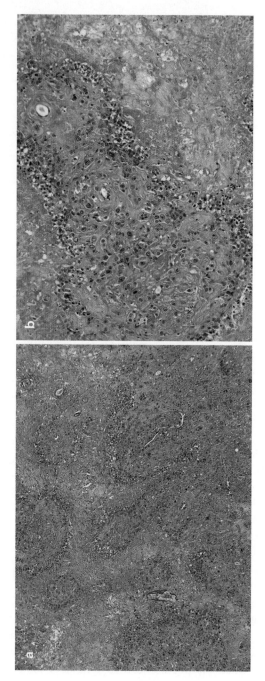

**Fig. 8.6** Epithelioid trophoblastic tumor. Note the expansile proliferation with cohesive tumor nests with (**a**, H.E. ×40), medium size intermediate trophoblastic cells with clear cytoplasm and hyalinized degenerative materials inside and outside of tumor nests (**b**, H.E. ×200)

very difficult to distinguish the two entities in a small biopsy or curettage specimen. Unlike PSTT, exaggerated placental site reaction does not form a mass lesion. Concurrent gestation or molar pregnancy, histologically evenly distributed multinucleated intermediate trophoblasts, and very low Ki-67 labeling (less than 1%) are features of exaggerated placental site reaction.

## 8.7  Placental Site Nodule

Placental site nodule (PSN) is retained placental chorionic laeve tissue, which persists for months or years after pregnancy. It is usually an inciden-tal microscopic finding and is not accompanied by serum hCG elevation. Histologically, PSN is a nodular or plaque-like lesion that is paucicel-lular with marked hyalinization and scattered inactive intermediate trophoblasts (Fig. 8.8). The main differential diagnosis is ETT. The absence of mass lesion, the presence of generally degenerative appearance and low-level of Ki-67 labeling index (below 10%) are features in sepa-rating PSN from ETT. Occasional lesions of PSN may show intermediate features in lesional size, cellularity, mitotic activity or Ki-67 index and therefore, a diagnosis of atypical PSN has been suggested, although the behavior of such lesion appears benign.

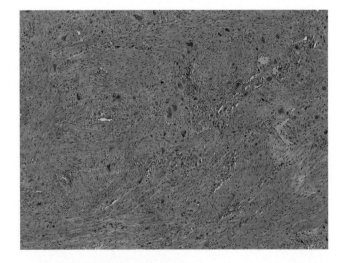

**Fig. 8.7** Exaggerate placental site reaction consists of an exuberant proliferation of implantation site intermediate trophoblasts involving the superficial myometrium. Note the presence of relatively evenly distributed multinucleated intermediate trophoblasts (H.E. ×40)

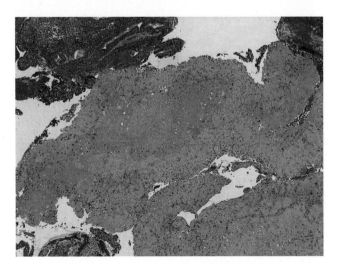

**Fig. 8.8** Placental site nodule shows hyalinized nodules or plaques with scattered intermediate trophoblasts (H.E. ×40)

## Suggested Reading

Berkowitz RS, Goldstein DP. Molar pregnancy. N Engl J Med 2009;360:1639–1645.

Buza N, Hui P. Gestational Trophoblastic Diseases: Histological Diagnosis in the Molecular Era (invited review). Diagnostic Histopathology. 2010, Sep 17. [Epub ahead of print]

Fox H, Sebire NJ. Pathology of the placenta. 3rd Edn. Saunders, Philadelphia, PA. 2007.

Lipata F, et al. Precise DNA genotyping diagnosis of hydatidiform mole. Obstet Gynecol 2010;1115: 784–794.

Shih IM, Mazur MT, Kurman RJ. Gestational trophoblastic disease and related lesions. In: Kurman RJ (eds). Blaustein's pathology of the female genital tract. New York: Springer Verlag; 2002:1193–1224.

# Chapter 9
# Tumors of Fallopian Tube and Broad Ligament

**Keywords** Fallopian tube • Carcinoma

## 9.1 Benign Tumors and Tumor-Like Conditions

Endometrial polyp is the most frequent tumor-like condition, involving usually the first segment of the fallopian tube and resulting in infertility and ectopic pregnancy. Salpingitis, either acute or chronic, can cause tubal enlargement and pelvic symptoms. Long-term chronic salpingitis may result in cystic alterations and tubo-ovarian adhesion. Salpingitis isthmica nodosa is a bilateral nodular lesion mostly involving the isthmus. The lesion consists of diverticuli of the tubal mucosa associated with smooth muscle hypertrophy (Fig. 9.1). Adenomatoid tumor is the most common benign tumor of the fallopian tube. Rare benign tumors of the fallopian tube or broad ligament resemble their counterparts of ovarian primaries, including various cystadenomas and borderline tumors (serous, mucinous, and mixed). Endometriosis frequently involves the serosa of the fallopian tube and/or broad ligament. An abnormal extension of the endometrium into the mucosa of the fallopian tube (mucosal endometriosis) may lead to infertility or tubal pregnancy. Endocervical mucinous metaplasia may be associated with Peutz–Jeghers syndrome. Metaplastic papillary "tumor" is an incidental mucinous papillary lesion associated with a pregnancy. Ectopic adrenal rest is a relatively common finding in the broad ligament. Leiomyoma may involve the broad ligament and occasionally the fallopian tube.

## 9.2 Malignant Epithelial Tumors

Carcinomas of the fallopian tube represent less than 1% of all cancers of the female genital tract, and have a strong association with some inherited cancer syndromes (BRAC-1 and BRAC-2 germline mutation), particularly in a young patient. Most BRCA mutations related tubal carcinomas involve the fimbrium, and frequently are bilateral. Recent studies have indicated that distal tubal carcinomas, particularly intramucosal serous carcinomas, are frequently found in patients with a synchronous ovarian carcinoma.

Serous carcinoma is the most common histological type (>70%), followed by endometrioid carcinoma and malignant mullerian mixed tumor. They have similar histological and cytological characteristics to their endometrial or ovarian counterparts (Fig. 9.2a, b). Serous intraepithelial carcinoma is frequently present adjacent to an invasive tubal serous carcinoma (Fig. 9.3), and may be an incidental finding in a prophylactic salpingo-oophorectomy specimen of a BRCA mutation patient. p53 signature, a proposed precursor lesion of in situ serous carcinoma, may show focal moderate tubal epithelial atypia and overexpression of p53, but limited Ki-67 proliferative activity. A diagnosis of primary tubal carcinoma can be established when the epicenter of the tumor is tubal and there is evidence of

D. Chhieng and P. Hui (eds.), *Cytology and Surgical Pathology of Gynecologic Neoplasms*,
Current Clinical Pathology, DOI 10.1007/978-1-60761-164-6_9,
© Springer Science+Business Media, LLC 2011

**Fig. 9.1** Salpingitis isthmica
nodosa. Note the presence of
diverticuli of the tubal mucosa
associated with hypertrophy of
smooth muscle (H.E. ×40)

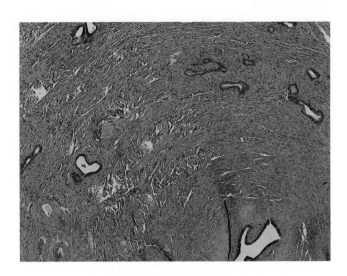

associated in situ carcinoma. However, such distinction can be difficult in some cases when a synchronous ovary or endometrial carcinoma is present. A mucosal colonization by endometrial or ovarian serous carcinoma is sometime impossible to be distinguished from a bona fide tubal carcinoma.

Female adnexal tumor of probable wolffian (mesonephric) origin (FATWO) is a distinct neoplasm of the broad ligament (most cases) and the fallopian tube. The tumor is seen in a wide range of age. Grossly, the tumor is unilateral, solid and nodular, gray-white to yellow. Histologically, the tumor consists of uniform small to medium size epithelioid cells with scanty eosinophilic cytoplasm. They form closely packed round to oval glands and tubules, imparting sieve-like appearance, and may be solid sheet in some areas (Fig. 9.4). Luminal accumulation of eosinophilic secretion may be present. The tumor cells are positive for cytokeratin, calretinin, vimentin, and CD10, but are negative for EMA and CEA. The tumor is considered to have a low malignant potential and up to 10% of the cases are clinically aggressive with pelvic spread and long-term recurrences.

Tubal teratomas, malignant lymphoma, ependymoma, and various sarcomas have been reported involving the fallopian tube and broad ligament.

Hydatidiform moles and placental site nodule occur in relation to an ectopic pregnancy. Tubal choriocarcinoma must be differentiated from a choriocarcinoma of the germ-cell origin.

## 9.3 Cytology

Adenocarcinomas originated from the fallopian tube may rarely present in cervicovaginal cytology. They should be suspected when cells diagnostic of adenocarcinoma are noted in a relatively clean background.

Since the most common histologic subtype is serous, the cytology typically consists of neoplastic cells arranged in small papillae or glandular structures. Individual cells demonstrate prominent nucleoli and cytoplasmic vacuoles. (Fig. 9.5) Psammoma bodies may be present, especially with well-differentiated carcinoma. The finding of psammoma bodies in gynecology

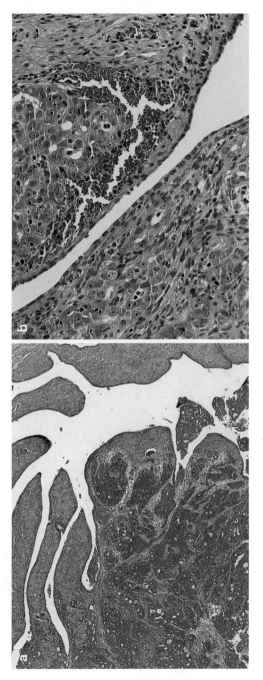

**Fig. 9.2** Tubal serous carcinoma. Low power (**a**, H.E. ×40) and high power (**b**, H.E. ×200)

**Fig. 9.3** Tubal intraepithelial
serous carcinoma (H.E. ×200)

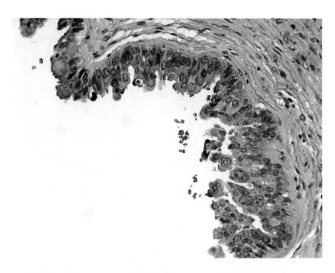

**Fig. 9.4** Female adnexal tumor
of probable wolffian origin. Note
the closely packed round to oval
glands and tubules, imparting
sieve-like appearance and the
presence of luminal accumulation
of eosinophilic secretion
(H.E. ×100)

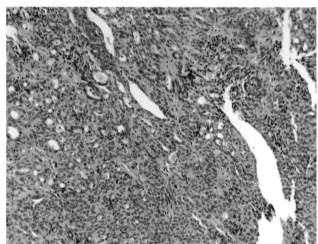

**Fig. 9.5** Fallopian tube
carcinoma. Papillary group of
atypical glandular cells with high
N:C ratio, prominent nucleoli,
and cytoplasmic vacuoles
(SurePath, Papanicolaou, ×400)

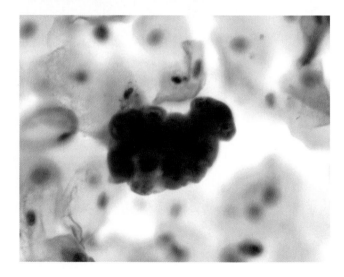

cytology is rare, accounting <0.001% of all Pap tests. The majority of cases are associated with benign conditions; the frequency of malignancy ranges from 0 to 20%.

## Suggested Reading

R.J. Kurman. Blaustein's Pathology of the Female Genital Tract. 5th Edition. Springer, Berlin, 2002.

# Chapter 10
# Epithelial Neoplasms of Ovary

Keywords  Ovary • Classification • Epithelial • Carcinoma • Metastases • Fine needle aspiration

## 10.1  General Classification of Ovarian Neoplasms

Primary ovarian tumors are generally classified according to their assumed cell origins into surface epithelial tumors, germ cell tumors, and tumors of sex-cord differentiation. Surface epithelial tumors are further subtyped into serous, mucinous, endometrioid, clear cell, and transitional cell tumors. Based on histological complexity, atypicality, invasiveness, and clinical behaviors, each subtype is further stratified into benign, borderline (atypical proliferative) and malignant categories (Table 10.1). Germ cell tumors encompass all histological subtypes found in male testis. Sex-cord tumors are named based on their cell differentiation: granulosa cells, theca cells, Sertoli cells, Leydig cells, and ovarian stromal cells. Secondary tumors represent 5% of all ovarian neoplasms with intestinal, appendiceal, gastric, and breast primaries as the most frequent sources of metastasis. The current chapter discusses primary and secondary epithelial tumors of the ovary (Table 10.1). However, clinicopathological staging discussed at the end of this chapter covers all types of primary ovarian neoplasms.

## 10.2  Primary Epithelial Ovarian Neoplasms

*Serous epithelial tumors* are the most common ovarian neoplasms (>30%), most of which are benign cystadenomas (60%). Borderline and carcinomas account for 15 and 25%, respectively.

1. *Serous cystadenomas* are cystic lesions with one or more cysts that are larger than 1 cm and contain serous fluid. The cyst lining is entirely smooth or with focal polypoid projections. The epithelial lining is simple, unstratified tubal or nonspecific epithelial types (Fig. 10.1). Papillae, if present, have broad bases and polypoid. The presence of significant fibrous stroma justifies a diagnosis of serous cystadenofibroma.

2. *Serous borderline tumors* are diagnosed in women of the reproductive age in most cases. The tumors are usually multilocular cystic mass with an average of 10 cm in size and are bilateral in about 40% of the cases. The cysts may contain serous or mucinous fluid. The cyst line is rough with gross complex papillae. Histologically, the tumor is characterized by the presence of complex hierarchical papillae, which are covered by stratified epithelial cells. Surface tumor cell tufting, budding, and exfoliating are present invariably (Fig. 10.2a). The tumor cells are polygonal to cuboidal with scant to abundant eosinophilic cytoplasm,

D. Chhieng and P. Hui (eds.), *Cytology and Surgical Pathology of Gynecologic Neoplasms,*
Current Clinical Pathology, DOI 10.1007/978-1-60761-164-6_10,
© Springer Science+Business Media, LLC 2011

**Table 10.1** Classification of epithelial ovarian tumors

| Major category | Subheading | Subtype or variant | Subtype or variant | Subtype or variant |
|---|---|---|---|---|
| Surface epithelial tumors | Serous tumors | Cystadenoma/ cystadenofibroma | Borderline serous tumor | Serous carcinoma |
| | Mucinous tumors | Cystadenoma/ cystadenofibroma | Borderline mucinous tumor | Mucinous carcinoma |
| | Endometrioid tumors | Cystadenoma/ cystadenofibroma | Borderline endometrioid tumor | Endometrioid carcinoma |
| | Clear cell tumors | Cystadenoma/ cystadenofibroma | Borderline clear cell tumor | Clear cell carcinoma |
| | Transitional cell tumors | Brenner tumor | Borderline Brenner tumor | Malignant Brenner and transitional cell carcinoma |
| | Mixed tumors | Benign | Borderline | Malignant |
| | Undifferentiated carcinomas | | | |
| Tumors of indefinite cell origin | Small cell carcinoma of hypercalcemic type | | | |
| | Small cell carcinoma of pulmonary type | | | |
| | Female adnexal tumor of probable wolffian origin | | | |
| | Hepatoid carcinoma | | | |
| Secondary carcinomas | | | | |

**Fig. 10.1** Serous cystadenoma. Note the simple unstratified epithelial cells (H.E. ×40)

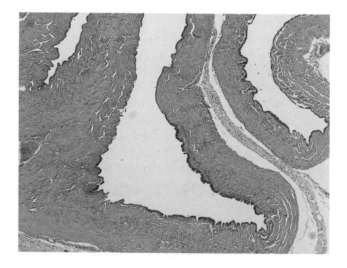

and do not contain significant mucin. Mild to moderate cytological atypia should be present in every case (Fig. 10.2b). Psammoma bodies are usually present. Small focus of serous tumor with the above borderline features in an otherwise cystadenoma has been referred to focally proliferative serous cystadenoma. However, more than 10% of the tumor with the borderline component or minor borderline growth involving the serosal surface of the ovary justifies a diagnosis of borderline serous tumor.

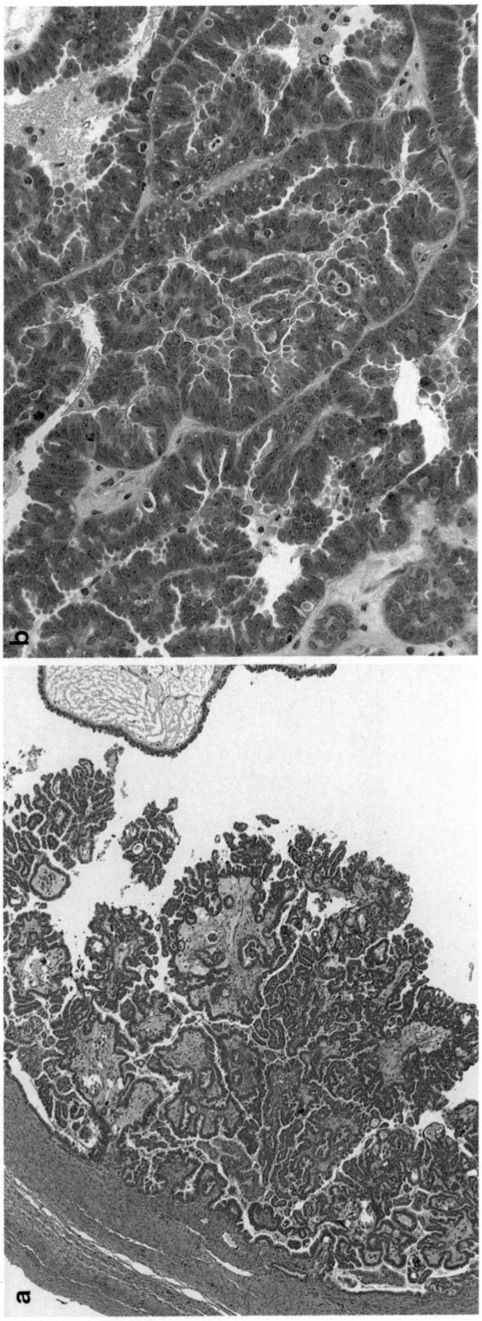

**Fig. 10.2** Serous borderline tumor. Low power view (**a**, H.E. ×40) and high power view (**b**, H.E. ×200). Note the surface tumor cell tufting, budding, exfoliating and mild to moderate cytological atypia

Focal marked cytological atypia with active mitosis, including the atypical mitosis justifies a diagnosis of intraepithelial carcinoma, and additional sampling of the tumor specimen should be performed to rule out a frank invasive carcinoma. Microinvasion is defined by the presence of less than 3 mm or 10 mm$^2$ in size of stromal invasion by single, small nest or papillae of more eosinophilic tumor cells. Micropapillary and cribriform serous borderline tumors are defined by the presence of at least 5 mm in size of nonbranching filiform micropapillae that are five times longer than their width, and tumor growth in cribriform patterns, respectively (Fig. 10.3). The cells of both micropapillary and cribriform tumors are more uniform in size and are mildly to moderately atypical.

Extraovarian tumor implants are present in more than one-third of serous borderline tumors, and divided into noninvasive and invasive forms. Noninvasive implants are tumor deposits on surface of pelvic organs with (desmoplastic noninvasive implant) or without desmoplastic response. Such implants may tract along the septum of the fat lobules and do not disturb the overall architecture of the organ (Fig. 10.4). Invasive implants are seen in 15% of serous borderline tumors. These implants are irregular

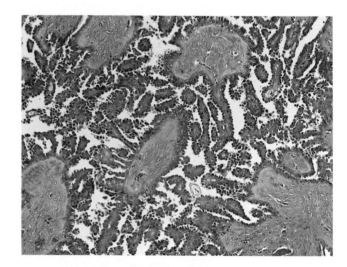

**Fig. 10.3** Serous borderline tumor with micropapillary pattern. Note the presence of nonbranching filiform micropapillae (H.E. ×100)

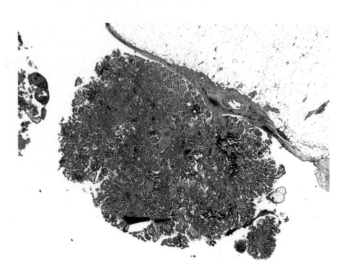

**Fig. 10.4** Noninvasive implant of serous borderline tumor. Note the undisturbed fat lobules (H.E. ×40)

tumor nests or papillae with disruption or invasion into the underlining normal tissue structures, such as fat lobules (Fig. 10.5). Micropapillary or cribriform serous borderline tumors are associated with higher rate of microinvasion and invasive implants. The presence of micropapillary or cribriform tumor deposits is considered invasive implants even in the absence of destructive invasion by some authors. Serous borderline tumors are frequently associated with endosalpingiosis involving various pelvic organs, including the lymph nodes. Endosalpingiosis should be separated from authentic tumor involvement either as implants or metastasis.

The overall prognosis of serous borderline tumor is excellent with 95% overall survival. Microinvasion, micropapillary/cribriform growth pattern, and invasive implants are adverse factors affecting the overall survival. In fact, many clinically aggressive tumors recur with transformation into well-differentiated serous carcinoma, particularly from micropapillary borderline tumors, although a subset may represent de novo serous carcinoma.

3. *Serous carcinomas* are divided into high-grade and low-grade tumors. They have distinct clinical and pathological characteristics, and recent investigation suggest that they are also different in their molecular pathogenesis. High-grade serous carcinoma is much more common and occurs in late reproductive and postmenopausal women. Histologically, most tumors are obviously invasive with papillary, cystic papillary to solid with slit-like space growth patterns, and markedly atypical cells, indistinguishable from those of endometrial serous carcinoma (Fig. 10.6a, b). Psammoma bodies are frequently present. Some high-grade serous tumors may have minor foci of anaplastic changes, cystic glands containing mucin, focal squamous differentiation, or focal trophoblastic differentiation. A separation from a primary peritoneal high-grade serous carcinoma relies on the finding of at least 5 mm ovarian parenchymal involvement to qualify for an ovarian primary. The tumor cells are typically positive for WT-1, P53, and P16, but none is absolutely specific regarding its diagnostic separation from an endometrial primary. Low-grade serous carcinomas are subdivided into psammoma carcinoma and well-differentiated micropapillary carcinoma. Psammoma carcinoma is defined as an invasive serous tumor consisting of low-grade cells, no solid tumor cell aggregates with more than 15 cells in any dimension, and more than 75% of tumor nests containing psammoma bodies (Fig. 10.7). Micropapillary serous carcinomas are associated with and likely arising from a micropapillary serous borderline tumor in at least 60% of the cases. They have uniform tumor cells with mild nuclear atypia (Fig. 10.8).

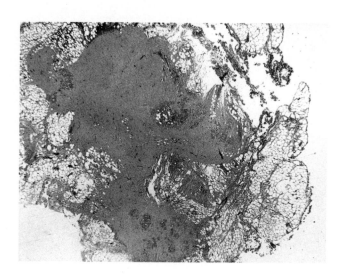

**Fig. 10.5** Invasive implant of serous borderline tumor (H.E. ×20)

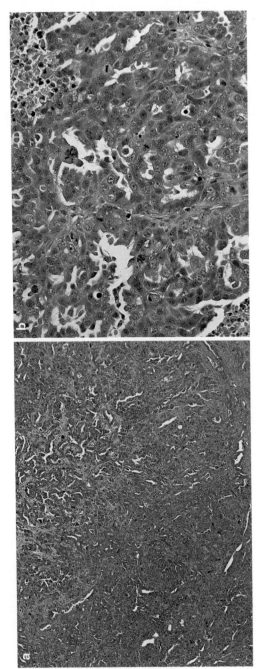

**Fig. 10.6** High grade ovarian serous carcinoma. Note the papillary, cystic papillary to solid with slit-like space growth patterns (**a**, H.E. ×40) and markedly atypical cells (**b**, H.E. ×200)

**Fig. 10.7** Psammoma carcinoma. Note the low grade carcinoma cells without solid tumor cell growth and more than 75% of tumor nests containing psammoma bodies (H.E. ×40)

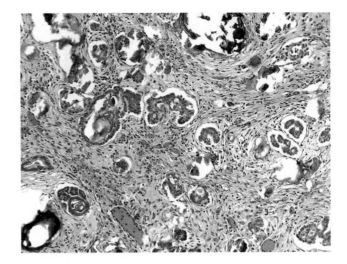

**Fig. 10.8** Well-differentiated serous carcinoma. This low-grade serous carcinoma is frequently associated with an ovarian micropapillary or cribriform serous borderline tumor (H.E. ×100)

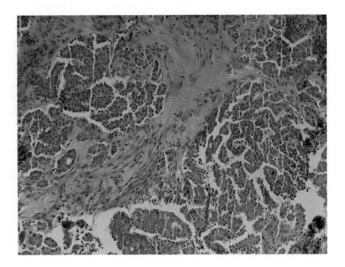

*Mucinous epithelial tumors* account for 15% of ovarian neoplasm, of which 80% are benign cystadenomas, 15% are borderline tumors, and less than 5% are carcinomas. Overall, 85% mucinous tumors are intestinal mucinous type and 15% are endocervical type. These are largest ovarian tumors on average and gross examination cannot reliably distinguish borderline tumors from carcinomas. They are unilateral in over 90% of the cases and often multicystic and contain mucinous fluid. Bilateral mucinous carcinoma should prompt a rigorous examination to rule out metastatic GI or pancreatic primary.

1. *Mucinous cystadenomas* are large and contain cystic glands lined by monolayer of benign columnar cells containing mucin with scattered goblet cells (Fig. 10.9). Simple papillary structures are usually present. Some tumors may have significant fibrous stroma (mucinous cystadenofibroma). Rupture of the glands may provoke a histiocytic response with multinucleated giant cells (mucinous granuloma). An otherwise mucinous cystadenoma with minor foci (<10%) of significant epithelial stratification and mild to moderate nuclear atypia should be diagnosed as "mucinous cystadenoma with focal atypia."

**Fig. 10.9** Mucinous cystadeoma
(H.E. ×40)

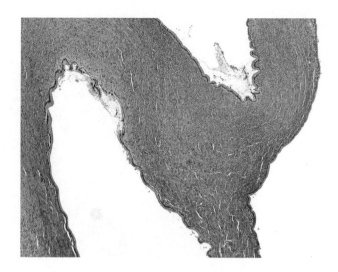

**Fig. 10.10** Mucinous borderline
tumor, intestinal type. Note the
complex papillation with
hierarchical branching of
stratified atypical mucinous
epithelium (H.E. ×40)

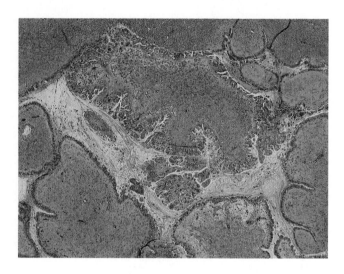

2. *Mucinous borderline tumor of the intestinal type* is multicystic and large with an average patient's age of 35 to 50 years. Microscopically, the cystic lining consists of complex papillation with hierarchical branching of stratified atypical mucinous epithelium (Fig. 10.10). Goblet cells are interspersed and sometimes numerous. The tumor cells generally have mild to moderate nuclear atypia. Stromal microinvasion is defined as no more than 3 or 5 mm size of invasive tumor nest, papillae, or single tumor cells with similar degrees of cytological atypia to the adjacent borderline tumor (Fig. 10.11). The presence of noninvasive foci of severe cytological atypia in an otherwise mucinous borderline tumor justifies a diagnosis of intraepithelial carcinoma. Microinvasive carcinoma is diagnosed when microscopic invasion consists of higher grade of tumor cells with severe cytological atypia. The presence of both microinvasive borderline tumor and microinvasive carcinoma should prompt a thorough examination of the specimen to rule out flank invasive mucinous carcinoma. *Mucinous borderline tumor of the endocervical type (seromucinous borderline tumor)* occurs in a younger patient group (35–40 years on average), and is frequently associated with endometriosis. They are often unilocular and smaller in size

**Fig. 10.11** Mucinous borderline
tumor with microinvasion
(H.E. ×100)

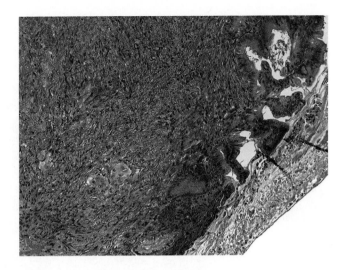

than the intestinal type tumor. The histological architectures of an endocervical type mucinous borderline tumor are similar to those of a serous borderline tumor, including cellular stratification, hierarchical branching of papillae, surface tufting and budding. The epithelial linings are usually mixed endocervical type and serous type (Fig. 10.12a, b). The presence of inflammatory cells, particular neutrophils, is characteristic. In contrast to the intestinal-type mucinous tumors (see below), seromucinous tumors express frequently ER, PR, but less WT-1, and are negative for CK20 and CDX2. They also have a much better prognosis than its intestinal counterpart.

3. *Mucinous carcinoma* has similar gross appearance of a borderline tumor and is diagnosed by histological findings of one of the two invasive growth patterns: expansile and infiltrative. Expansile invasion is characterized by complex glandular or papillary proliferations of highly atypical cells in cribriform or glandular arrangements with little or no intervening stroma (Fig. 10.13). A size of at least 3 or 5 mm is required to separate an expansile invasion from an intraepithelial carcinoma in a borderline tumor. Infiltrative invasion is characterized by stromal invasion by irregular tumor glands, nests or single cells along with a desmoplastic stromal response (Fig. 10.14). The tumor cells of mucinous carcinomas may have minimal to obvious mucin production

and goblet cells may or may not be present. Primary ovarian mucinous carcinomas should be separated from metastatic carcinomas, particularly if the tumor is bilateral, necrotic or with signet ring cell features. Primary ovarian mucinous carcinomas are immunoreactive to CK7 with or without CK20. However, tumor arising from an ovarian terotoma may have an immunophenotype of that of colonic adenocarcinomas. CDX-2 is positive in a third of the cases. Rare mucinous carcinoma of the endocervical type occurs in association with seromucinous borderline tumor, and the diagnosis requires at least 5 mm stromal invasion.

Mucinous ovarian tumors may develop sarcoma-like mural nodules in rare cases. These are intracystic, fleshy and solid nodules, and sharply demarcated from the mucinous epithelial tumor tissue grossly and microscopically. The lesion consists of mixed spindle and histiocytoid cells that may demonstrate marked pleomorphism and active mitosis. Various amount of inflammatory cells, extravasated red cells and osteoclastic-like histiocytes are characteristically present (Fig. 10.15). Hemorrhage and necrosis are also common. Sarcoma-like mural nodules are reactive in nature and should be separated from the anaplastic carcinomatous nodule in a poorly differentiated carcinoma or the sarcoma component in a malignant mixed mullerian tumor.

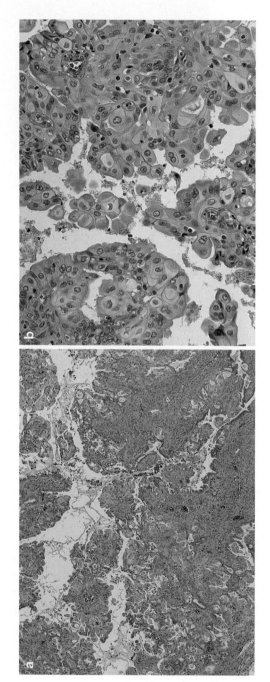

**Fig. 10.12** Mucinous borderline tumor of endocervical type. Note mixed endocervical type and serous type tumor cells and the presence of inflammatory cells. Low power view (**a**, H.E. ×40) and high power view (**b**, H.E. ×200)

**Fig. 10.13** Mucinous
adenocarcinoma with
expansile invasion (H.E. ×20)

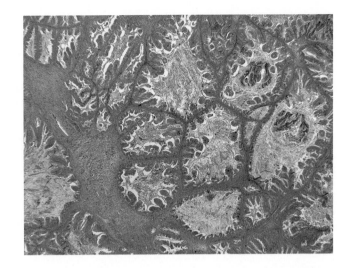

**Fig. 10.14** Mucinous
adenocarcinoma with
destructive invasion (H.E. ×40)

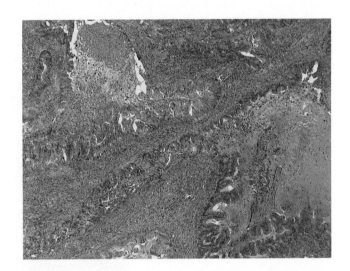

**Fig. 10.15** Sarcomatoid mural
nodule. Note the mixed spindle
and histiocytoid cells that have
marked pleomorphism and active
mitotic activity (H.E. ×200)

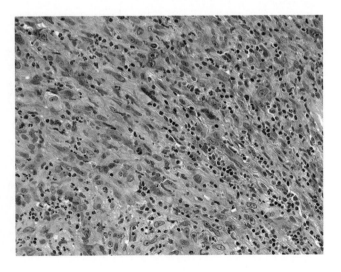

*Endometrioid epithelial tumors* roughly represents 5% of all ovarian tumors, but endometrioid adenocarcinomas account for 15% of all ovarian epithelial malignancies. They are often associated with ovarian or pelvic endometriosis and may have similar pathogenesis with that of the endometrial endometrioid adenocarcinoma. Grossly, these tumors are similar to other types of ovarian epithelial tumors, although more often associated with cystic ovarian endometriosis with hemorrhage. Endometrioid cystadenoma is essentially cystic endometriosis with less or no endometrial stromal component. Significant fibromatous component is seen in an endometri-oid cystadenofibroma. Endometrioid borderline tumors are cystic proliferation of proliferative endometrial glands with an overall histological appearance seen in the uterine endometrial hyperplasia with or without cytological atypia (Fig. 10.16). The presence of high-grade dysplasia justifies "endometrioid borderline tumor with intraepithelial carcinoma." Endometrioid carcinoma of the ovary can display all histological variations seen in uterine endometrioid carcinomas (Fig. 10.17). Squamous differentiation is common. Coexistence with endometrioid borderline tumor with morphological transition is a helpful hint for diagnosis (Fig. 10.18).

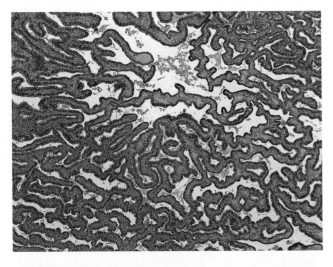

**Fig. 10.16** Endometrioid borderline tumor. Note the overall histological appearance similar to that of complex endometrial hyperplasia (H.E. ×40)

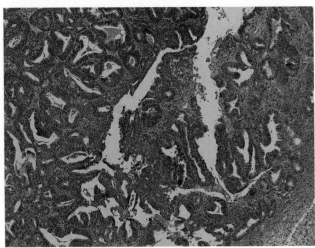

**Fig. 10.17** Endometrioid adenocarcinoma (H.E. ×40)

**Fig. 10.18** Endometrioid adenocarcinoma associated with endometriosis (H.E. ×40)

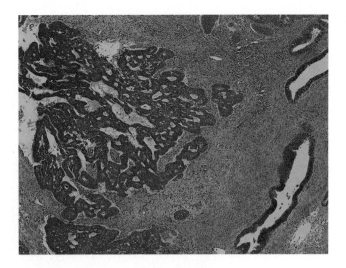

**Table 10.2** Differential diagnosis of histological similar tumors involving both ovary and endometrium

| Ovarian primary | Endometrial primary | Synchronous tumors |
|---|---|---|
| Larger parenchymal ovarian tumor | Dominant endometrial tumor and ovarian surface implants | Superficial or nonmyoinvasive endometrial tumor and ovarian parenchymal tumor |
| Ovarian endometriosis and/or pelvic endometriosis | Atypical endometrial hyperplasia | Atypical endometrial hyperplasia and ovarian endometriosis |
| Direct extension into myometrium by ovarian tumor | Deep myometrial invasion by endometrial tumor | No ovarian tumor extension to myometrium |
| Unilateral ovarian tumor | Bilateral ovarian tumors | Unilateral ovarian tumor |
| Peritoneal spreading pattern and no lymphovascular involvement, particularly hilum of the ovary | Lymphovascular spreading involving uterine wall and hilum of the ovary | Absence of lymphovascular invasion and no evidence of extraovarian tumor spreading |

Endometrioid adenocarcinomas of the ovary are graded into well, moderately and poorly differentiated according to the percentage of solid growth pattern and nuclear grade. Differential diagnoses include endometrioid yolk sac tumor, Sertoli–Leydig cell tumor, tumor of probable wolffian origin, ovarian ependymoma, and metastatic adenocarcinomas. Synchronous and metachronous uterine endometrioid carcinomas are frequently encountered diagnostic challenges. When histologically similar tumors involving both endometrium and ovary, the presence of unilateral, larger ovarian parenchymal tumor, and findings of ovarian endometriosis favor an ovarian primary or synchronous ovarian tumor (Table 10.2).

*Clear cell tumors* account for less than 5% of ovarian neoplasms. Benign and borderline clear cell tumors are adenofibromatous in almost every case and are rare. In contrast, clear cell carcinomas are relatively common and are the most frequent tumor associated with endometriosis among all ovarian cancers. Clear cell adenofibroma consists of significant fibrous component with scattered glands lined by clear, flattened nonatypical epithelial cells. Mild nuclear atypia justifies a diagnosis of borderline clear cell tumor (Fig. 10.19a, b). Focal stromal invasion of less than 3–5 mm size can be interpreted as microinvasive clear cell borderline tumor. A clear cell tumor with significant cytological atypia is clear cell carcinoma until proven otherwise.

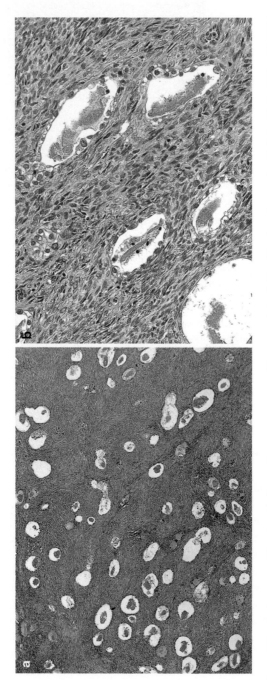

**Fig. 10.19** Clear cell borderline tumor. Note the significant fibrous component with scattered glands lined by clear, flattened epithelial cells (**a**, H.E. ×40). Mild nuclear atypia justifies a diagnosis of borderline clear cell tumor (**b**, H.E. ×200)

The epithelial components of a clear cell carcinoma may be tubocystic, glands, papillae, tubules, or solid. Polygonal or cuboidal tumor cells with clear cytoplasm are typical findings, so as hobnail cells that have apically located hyperchromatic nuclei (Fig. 10.20a, b). The stroma of the tumor is characteristically hyalinized, and sometimes colloidal. Oxyphilic clear cell carcinomas have more solid nests of cells with abundant eosinophilic cytoplasm. Rare clear cell carcinomas have signet ring cells in singles or solid sheets with cytoplasmic mucin production (Fig. 10.21). Clear cell carcinoma is a high-grade malignancy. Although clear cell adenofibroma and borderline tumor are benign, even with microinvasion, they need to be sampled thoroughly to rule out the coexistence of clear cell carcinoma.

*Transitional cell tumors* account for less than 2% of ovarian neoplasms. Benign Brenner tumor is the most common and frequently an incidental finding. The tumor consists of dense fibromatous stroma with scattered round to oval solid epithelial nests with or without punctate round cysts that may be filled with eosinophilic secretion (Fig. 10.22). The epithelial lining consists of oval to elongated cells that have nuclear grooves and pale cytoplasm. Mucinous differentiation may be present in the forms of glands or mucinous epithelium lining the cystic tumor nests. Borderline Brenner tumors have predominant epithelial proliferation over stromal component. They resemble a low-grade urothelial carcinoma with noninvasive papillary growth and low nuclear grade (Fig. 10.23). Malignant Brenner tumors are invasive carcinomas of either transitional or squamous type in association with an identifiable Brenner tumor or borderline Brenner tumor (Fig. 10.24). Transitional carcinoma is an invasive cystic tumor without identifiable Brenner tumor component. It resembles a high-grade urothelial carcinoma with undulating, broad nonbranching papillae (Fig. 10.25). The tumor cells are relatively uniform with round to elongated nuclei with moderate to high atypicality and numerous mitosis. Mixed carcinomatous components are frequently present, including serous, endometrioid, mucinous, or clear cell. The tumor cells express WT-1 and uroplakin III but CK20. Brenner tumor and borderline Brenner tumor are benign. Transitional cell carcinomas are highly aggressive tumor with high stage presentation in 70% of the cases, comparing with 20% in malignant Brenner tumor cases.

## 10.3 Ovarian Epithelial Tumors of Uncertain Origin

*Small cell carcinoma of hypercalcemic type* is a highly aggressive tumor of young patients with an average age of 24 years. Although qualified by its name, hypercalcemia is clinically absent in about 30% of the cases. The tumor is unilateral and frequently large. The cut surface is solid, fleshy, and white to tan. Hemorrhage and necrosis are common. Histologically, the tumor consists of diffuse proliferation of closely packed epithelial cells (Fig. 10.26a). In many cases, pseudofollicular cysts with eosinophilic fluid are present. The tumor has small cells with little cytoplasm, a hyperchromatic nucleus and distinct small nucleoli (Fig. 10.26b). Some cases may contain clusters of larger cells with abundant eosinophilic or rhabdoid cytoplasm. When such large cell component predominates, a diagnosis of large cell variant of small cell carcinoma of hypercalcemic type may be entertained. The typical immunohistochemical profile consists of cytokeratin+, NSE+, vimentin+, B72.3−, and S100−. A third of the tumors are also chromogranin+.

*Small cell carcinoma of pulmonary type* is a highly malignant epithelial tumor with essentially identical histology to that of the pulmonary counterpart. The patients are older. A diagnostic separation from small cell carcinoma of hypercalcemic type is made by its more closely packed cells with nuclear molding, salt-and-pepper chromatin pattern and inconspicuous nucleoli.

*Hepatoid carcinoma* is a rare tumor seen in postmenopausal women with elevated serum AFP. The tumor histologically resembles hepatocellular carcinoma by the presence of sheets and cords of large cells with abundant eosinophilic cytoplasm, round and centrally located nuclei. Mitosis and hyaline globules may be numerous. Cytoplasmic bile pigment may be found.

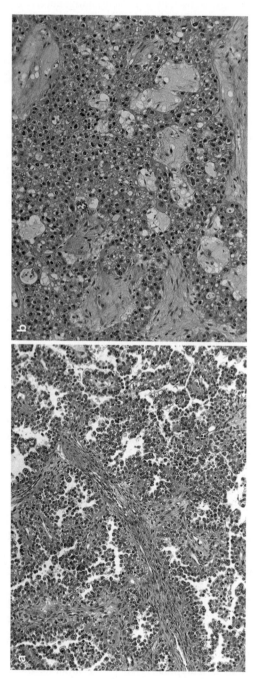

**Fig. 10.20** (**a**, **b**) Clear cell carcinoma. Note the papillae, tubules, or solid sheets of polygonal or cuboidal clear tumor cells and hobnail cells

**Fig. 10.21** Clear cell carcinomas with signet ring cells. Note the solid growth of tumor cells with clear or mucin containing cytoplasm and targetoid appearance in singles or solid sheets. Low power view (**a**, H.E. ×40) and high power view (**b**, H.E. ×200)

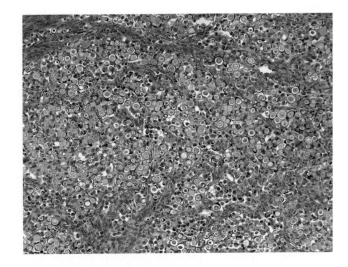

**Fig. 10.22** Brenner tumor (H.E. ×40)

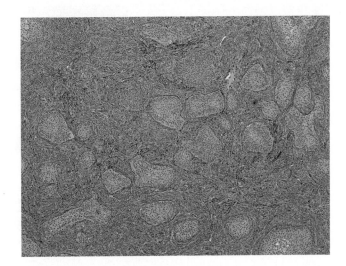

**Fig. 10.23** Borderline Brenner tumor. Note the overall resemblance to a low-grade urothelial carcinoma with noninvasive papillary growth pattern and low nuclear grade (H.E. ×40)

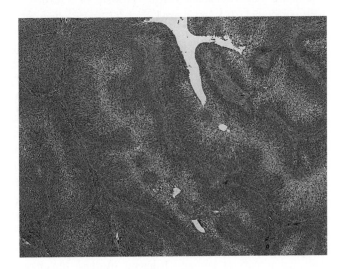

**Fig. 10.24** Malignant Brenner tumor (H.E. ×100). Benign Brenner tumor component is present elsewhere in the tumor

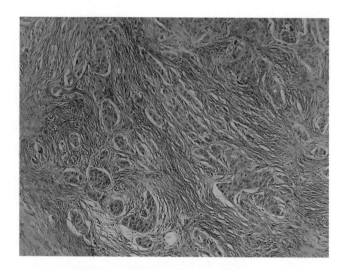

**Fig. 10.25** Transitional cell carcinoma. Note the overall resemblance to a high-grade urothelial carcinoma with undulating, broad nonbranching papillae (H.E. ×40)

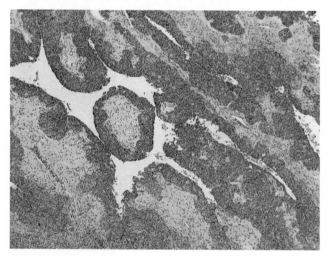

The tumor cells are characteristically positive for AFP, polyclonal CEA and Hepa-1.

*Female adnexal tumor of probable wolffian origin* occasionally occurs as a primary ovarian lesion. The tumor is unilateral and may be large. Its histology is described under uterine mesenchymal tumors (Chapter 9).

## 10.4  Secondary Carcinomas Involving Ovary

Ovary is a frequent target for metastatic carcinomas, particularly of the GI and breast primaries. They represent more than 5% of ovarian malignant epithelial tumors at surgery. Bilateral ovarian involvement, ovarian surface tumors, the presence of multiple discrete and heterogeneous parenchymal tumor nodules and the presence of lymphovascular tumor thrombi are common features of metastatic carcinoma. It is important to note that metastatic carcinomas may simulate a primary ovarian carcinoma by paradoxical metamorphosis, including maturation into a low-grade appearance, gross cystic appearance, microscopic follicle-like changes, and stromal luteinization. In rare occasions, the metastatic tumor may present before the primary carcinoma is clinical detectable. Generally, when an extraovarian carcinoma is present, every effort should be made to histologically compare with the ovarian tumor.

*Krukenberg tumor* is a bilateral, metastatic mucinous adenocarcinoma of the signet ring type.

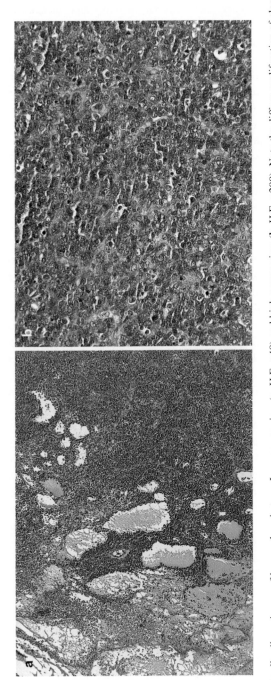

**Fig. 10.26** Small cell carcinoma of hypercalcemic type. Low power view (**a**, H.E. ×40) and high power view (**b**, H.E. ×200). Note the diffuse proliferation of closely packed small epithelial cells with little cytoplasm and hyperchromatic nuclei and the presence of pseudofollicular cysts with eosinophilic fluid

Over two-third of the cases, the primary tumor is a gastric signet ring cell carcinoma of the pylorus, typically in a young woman. Other primary sites include appendix, colon, pancreaticobillary tract and breast. Although most Krukenberg tumors are present with a prior diagnosis at the primary site, not uncommonly, an occult gastric carcinoma may only be found either some months or years after the ovarian tumor has been removed, or upon a careful autopsy examination. Krukenberg tumor may grossly and microscopically simulate fibroma or fibrothecoma. They are solid, firm to fleshy and mostly white to tan-yellow with vague nodularity. Histologically, the tumor diffusely involves ovaries with alternating edematous and cellular fibrothecomatous areas (Fig. 10.27a). Mucin-laden signet ring cells may be found as singles, small aggregates or forming nests (Fig. 10.27b). Mucin production is obvious or easily demonstrated by special stains. Small glands, tubular structure, or glands with squamous or endometrioid differentiation may be seen in rare cases as minor components. Immunostains may help to identify the primary tumors: gastric primary is positive for CDX2 and HerPar1, but negative for ER; colonic primary is positive for MUC2, MUC5, and CDX2 but negative for HerPar1 and ER; breast primary is positive for MUC1, CK7, and ER. Primary ovarian tumors that may mimic Krukenberg tumor include clear cell carcinoma with signet ring cell features and mucinous carcinoid tumors with signet ring cells. So-called primary Krukenberg tumor is likely a poorly differentiated mucinous carcinoid tumor arising from an ovarian teratoma. Krukenberg tumor may simulate some benign and reactive conditions, including fibrothecoma, massive ovarian edema, and mucicarminophilic histiocytosis.

*Colorectal carcinoma* is the most common source for metastasis and up to 80% are rectosigmoid primaries. Misinterpretation as ovarian primary occurs in half of the cases clinically or microscopically. The tumor involves one ovary in 40% of the cases. The tumor usually simulates an endometrioid adenocarcinoma microscopically. Features suggest a metastatic colonic carcinoma include (1) the presence of extensive tumor necrosis with accumulation of necrotic debris

(dirty necrosis, Fig. 10.28), (2) an adenocarcinoma with low "FIGO" grade (open glands) but severe cytological atypia (grade 3 nuclei and brisk mitotic activity) and nuclear stratification, and (3) an absence of squamous differentiation. Combination immunohistochemistry of CK7, CK20, and CDX-2 is very helpful in the differential diagnosis: colonic and appendiceal carcinomas are CK7− (80%), CK20+ (95%) and CDX-2+ (90–100%); gastric and pancreaticobillary carcinomas are CK7+ (80%), CK20+ (80–100%), and CDX-2 + (60–100%); primary ovarian endometrioid carcinomas are CK7+ (97–100%), CK20−(90–100%), and CDX-2− (100%); and primary ovarian mucinous carcinomas are CK7+ (100%), CK20+ (60%), and CDX-2+ (50%).

*Low-grade appendiceal mucinous tumors* (low grade mucinous neoplasm or low grade mucinous adenocarcinoma) involve ovary with an extensive mucin production (pseudomyxoma ovarii). Gross gelatinous appearance and microscopic dissecting mucin pools with highly differentiated mucinous epithelial cells are characteristic. Frequently associated with pseudomyxoma ovarii, pseudomyxoma peritonei is a clinical diagnosis and its presence essentially establishes an appendiceal primary mucinous tumor (Fig. 10.29).

*Carcinoid tumors* of GI tract, ileum as the most common, or lung can metastasize to ovary. They often present with carcinoid syndrome clinically. The microscopic growth patterns are insular (most common) or trebecular. Mucinous carcinoid tumors are almost always appendiceal primary. Bilateral involvement and the absence of teratomatous elements are supportive evidence of metastatic carcinoid tumor. Metastatic carcinoid tumor may present first clinically in rare cases, and the GI primary may not be evident until some months after the discovery of the ovarian tumor.

*Metastatic pancreaticobillary mucinous tumor or carcinomas* may greatly simulate an ovarian primary mucinous tumor grossly and microscopically. Bilateral involvement with nodular ovarian lesions, histological heterogeneity of tumor areas ranging from benign cystadenoma, borderline mucinous tumor to frankly

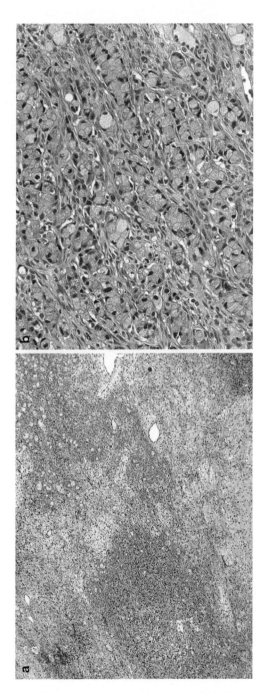

**Fig. 10.27** Krukenberg tumor. Note the alternating edematous and cellular fibrothecomatous areas (**a**, H.E. ×40) and mucin-laden signet ring cells as singles, small aggregates, or forming nests (**b**, H.E. ×200)

**Fig. 10.28** Metastatic colorectal
adenocarcinoma. Note the
extensive tumor necrosis with
accumulation of necrotic debris
(dirty necrosis) (H.E. ×40)

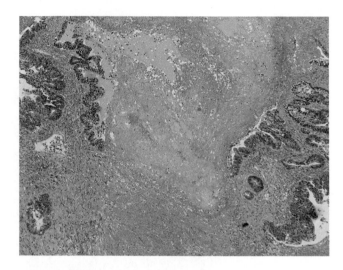

**Fig. 10.29** Pseudomyxoma
peritonei. Note the microscopic
dissecting mucin pools with
highly differentiated mucinous
epithelial cells (H.E. ×40)

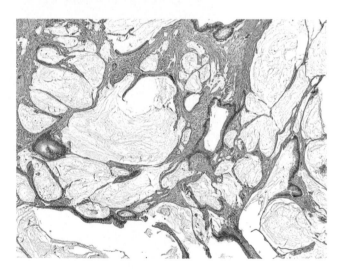

invasive adenocarcinomas (Fig. 10.30a, b) and
an immunohistochemical profile of CK20+,
CK7+, MUC5+, and Dpc4− are diagnostic features of these metastatic tumors.

*Breast carcinoma* is also a common source of
ovarian secondary tumor, although most are not
diagnostic challenging. Metastatic breast carcinomas are usually incidental findings with the
primary diagnosis well established in almost all
cases. Most are metastatic ductal carcinomas.
Breast lobular carcinomas may be interpreted as
granular cell tumor or carcinoid tumors, or
entirely missed due to their diffuse growth pattern and low nuclear grade. Both ovarian and
breast carcinomas are commonly positive for ER

and PR. GCDF-15 positivity is helpful marker
for the breast primary.

Rare metastatic renal cell carcinomas can
simulate ovarian clear cell carcinoma.
Monomorphism of the tumor cells, the absence
of hobnailing cells, the presence of intratumoral
hemorrhage, and sinusoidal vascular dilation are
helpful histological features of metastatic renal
clear cell carcinomas.

Metastatic urothelial carcinomas can be
separated from the ovarian transitional cell
tumors by clinical evaluation, the absence of
benign Brenner tumor component and an
immunohistochemical profile of CK7+, CK20+,
uroplakin+, and thrombomodulin+.

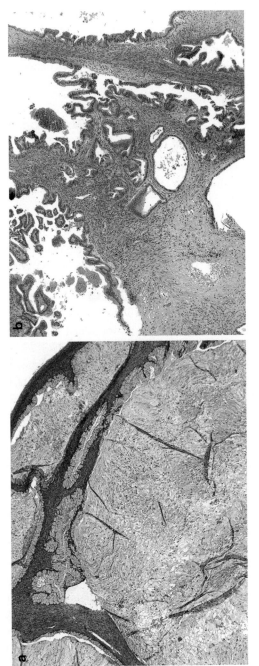

**Fig. 10.30** (**a, b**) Mucinous pancreatic adenocarcinoma metastasizing to ovary. Note the deceptively benign appearing mucin glands in some areas (H.E. ×40)

## 10.5 Cytology

### 10.5.1 Exfoliative Cytology in Pap Test

Similar to fallopian tube adenocarcinoma, ovarian carcinoma should be suspected when cells diagnostic of adenocarcinoma noted in a relatively clean background. The cytology is similar to that of endometrial adenocarcinoma. Cytoplasmic vacuoles are common but intracytoplasmic neutrophils are usually absent. The finding of papillary groups and psammoma bodies and the absence of tumor diathesis should raise the possibility of an ovarian primary.

### 10.5.2 Fine Needle Aspiration Biopsy

Until recently, the use of fine needle aspiration biopsy (FNA) in the preoperative management of patients with ovarian mass has not been widely accepted because of the concern of the possibility of spilling the contents of tumor into the peritoneal cavity. However, for women who desire to preserve ovarian function, FNA has been increasingly utilized for the diagnosis and treatment of nonneoplastic cystic lesions. Therefore, one of the major goals of ovarian FNA is to distinguish between nonneoplastic and neoplastic cystic lesions since the former may be treated conservatively while the latter will likely require surgical intervention. For patients with a prior ovarian malignancy, FNA is also indicated to rule out recurrent disease.

FNA of ovary may be performed via transvaginal and transabdominal route, usually under ultrasound guidance. In addition, FNA can be performed under direct vision during laparoscopy or laparotomy. Transrectal approach is seldom utilized because of the concern regarding infection. Sonographic criteria for identifying cysts that can be safely evaluated by FNA include size less than 10 cm in diameter, unilaterality, thin, smooth cyst wall and septa, hypovascular, low echogenicity, and the absence of ascites.

FNA is almost never performed for normal ovaries. Various normal epithelial and mesenchymal components may be picked up inadvertently by the needles. Depending on the sampling route, these components include squamous epithelium, colonic epithelium, mesothelium, fibroadipose tissue, and muscle. They should be considered as contaminants.

### 10.5.3 Nonneoplastic Cysts

#### 10.5.3.1 Follicular Cysts

Depending on the degree of maturation, the cellularity of follicular cysts can vary from scant to high. The background can be clean or hemorrhagic. The cellular component usually consists of predominantly granulose cells. The latter appear singly, loosely cohesive sheets, or three-dimensional clusters. They resemble histiocytes with small to abundant amount of foamy cytoplasm, round to oval nuclei, and small, distinct nucleoli (Fig. 10.31). Nuclear grooves and mitotic figures are sometimes noted. Atypical features such as very high cellularity, nuclear enlargement, high N:C ratio, prominent nucleoli, and frequent mitotic figures, raising the possibility of a malignancy. A benign diagnosis should favor when the atypical features are spotty and cells typical of granulose cells are present.

#### 10.5.3.2 Endometriosis

The cystic fluid appears brownish black. Cytologically, the predominant cellular component is hemosiderin-laden macrophages in a hemorrhagic background. A definitive diagnosis requires the identification of endometrial cells, which appear as variable size clusters of small cells with scanty cytoplasm and small, hyperchromatic nuclei (Figs. 10.32 and 10.33). However, endometrial cells are only present in some but not all endometriotic cysts. Endometrial stroma, which is immunoreactive with CD10, may rarely be observed, particularly in cell-block preparation.

**Fig. 10.31** Follicular cyst.
Cohesive cluster of granulose
cells with abundant amount of
granular to foamy cytoplasm,
uniform round to oval nuclei.
Distinct nucleoli are noted in
occasional cells (ThinPrep,
Papanicolaou, ×400)

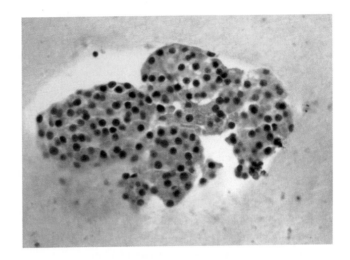

**Fig. 10.32** Endometriosis.
Crowded group of glandular cells
with mild atypia (ThinPrep,
Papanicolaou, ×400)

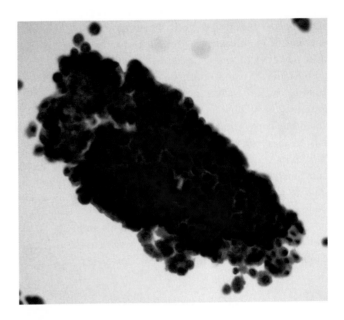

**Fig. 10.33** Endometriosis.
Numerous hemosiderin-laden
macrophages are also noted
(ThinPrep, Papanicolaou, ×400)

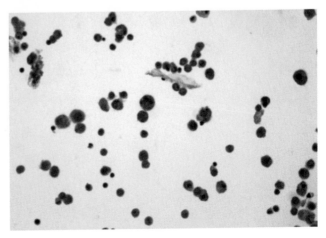

### 10.5.3.3 Neoplastic Ovarian Cysts

Cystic changes can occur in any histologic sub-types of ovarian neoplasms. Therefore, the following discussion is limited to the more common cystic ovarian tumors, including serous and mucinous ovarian tumors.

#### 10.5.3.3.1 Serous Tumors

Cytologic findings vary with the histologic grade of the tumors. Aspirates from serous cystadenoma and cystadenofibroma are usually of scant cellularity and consists of bland appearing cuboidal cells in cohesive clusters and sheets. Individual cells have moderate amount of nondescript cytoplasm, round to oval nuclei, and small nucleoli. Ciliated epithelial cells are occasionally noted (Fig. 10.34). Histiocytes are often present in the background. A diagnosis of cystadenofibroma should be considered when there is a conspicuous presence of fibroblasts.

Aspirates of serous borderline tumor usually contain papillary clusters of epithelial cells with mild to moderate cytologic atypia. Psammoma bodies may be present. It is impossible to differentiate between serous borderline tumor and well-differentiated serous papillary cystadenocarcinoma based on cytology alone because their separation depends on the evaluation of stromal invasion.

Serous papillary cystadenocarcinomas are seldom aspirated because their sonographic appearance usually does not meet the criteria for evaluating ovarian cysts using FNA. In the rare instances, the aspirates are cellular and composed of three-dimensional clusters and papillary groups of atypical epithelial cells. Necrosis is frequent and may be the predominant finding.

#### 10.5.3.3.2 Mucinous Tumors

Aspirates of mucinous tumors are characterized by the presence of tall columnar epithelial cells in a mucinous background. Individual cells demonstrate round to oval, often peripherally placed nuclei and cytoplasmic vacuolation (Fig. 10.35). Cytologic and nuclear atypia increases as the tumors progress from cystadenoma to borderline tumor to cystadenocarcinomas.

#### 10.5.3.3.3 Other Surface Epithelial Tumors

Other surface epithelial tumors, such as endometrioid and clear cell ovarian carcinomas and Brenners tumors, are seldom encountered in FNA of ovary. The former two usually demonstrate obviously malignant epithelial cells (Fig. 10.36). Brenners tumor is characterized by the presence

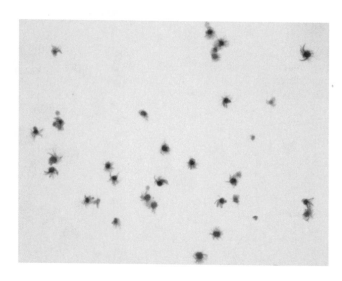

**Fig. 10.34** Serous cystadenoma. Bland discohesive cuboidal cells with cilia are noted (ThinPrep, Papanicolaous, ×400)

**Fig. 10.35** Mucinous cystadenoma. Papillary group of mucin producing columnar cells with basal-oriented, bland appearing nuclei. Scattered histiocytes are noted in the background (ThinPrep, Papanicolaou, ×400)

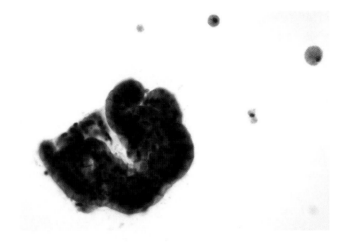

**Fig. 10.36** Ovarian carcinoma, high grade. Patient had a prior history of oophorectomy for ovarian carcinoma, now present with pelvic mass. Aspirate of FNA of the pelvic mass demonstrates syncytial group of highly pleomorphic epithelial cells (direct smear, Papanicolaou, ×400)

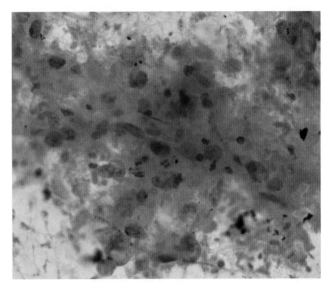

**Fig. 10.37** Colon carcinoma, metastatic to ovary. Cohesive group of pleomorphic columnar and epithelioid cells in a background of necrosis (direct smear, Diff-Quik, ×400)

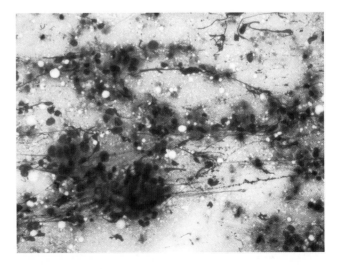

of relatively uniform cells with "coffee-bean" shaped nuclei and nuclear grooves.

### 10.5.3.3.4   Metastatic Tumors

Metastatic tumors usually present with bilateral ovarian involvement and do not usually meet the sonographic criteria for FNA. It is not surprising that there are only a few reports on the cytology of metastatic tumors in the ovary in the literature. The cytologic appearances in ovary are similar to those seen in other parts of the body (Fig. 10.37).

## Suggested Reading

Clement PB, Young RH. Atlas of Gynecologic Surgical Pathology. Saunders Publisher, Philadelphia, PA, 2008.

Kurman R. Blaustein's Pathology of the Female Genital Tract. 5th Edition. Springer, Berlin, 2002.

Mulvany NJ. (1996) Aspiration cytology of ovarian cysts and cystic neoplasms. A study of 235 aspirates. Acta Cytol. 40:911–20.

Prat J. Pathology of the Ovary. Saunders Publisher, Philadelphia, PA, 2004.

Papathanasiou K, et al. (2004) Fine needle aspiration cytology of the ovary: is it reliable? Clin. Exp. Obstet. Gynecol. 31:191–3.

# Chapter 11
# Nonepithelial Tumor of Ovary

**Keywords** Ovary • Nonepithelial • Germ cell tumors • Sex cord-stromal tumors

## 11.1 General Classification of Nonepithelial Ovarian Tumors

Nonepithelial ovarian tumors are generally grouped into germ cell tumors, sex cord-stromal tumors and varieties of miscellaneous tumors, including lymphomas and soft tissue tumors.

## 11.2 Ovarian Germ Cell Tumors

Ovarian germ cell tumors are neoplastic transformations of ovarian primitive oocyte and account for one-third of ovarian neoplasms. Over 95% are benign teratomas. Malignant immature germ cell tumors account for only 3% of all ovarian malignancies. While mature teratomas are seen in all age groups, malignant immature germ cell tumors are predominantly found in patients younger than 30 years of age. Classification of germ cell tumors is presented in Table 11.1.

*Teratomas* consist of tissue type(s) derived from one, two or three embryonic germ layers (ectoderm, endoderm, and mesoderm). Mature teratomas are further classified into mature cystic teratoma, mature solid teratoma, fetiform teratoma, and monodermal teratoma.

Mature cystic or solid teratomas may have all three embryonic tissue types in any combination, although ectodermal skin and its appendages are always present as dominant components. Ectodermal neuronal tissues (glia, cerebrum, cerebellum, choroid plexus, and retina) may be present in some cases (Fig. 11.1). Adipose tissue, smooth and skeletal muscle, teeth, bone, and cartilage are common mesodermal components. Endodermal differentiation is frequently represented by gastrointestinal, pulmonary, and thyroid tissues. So-called fetiform teratoma is a mature teratoma that has a gross resemblance to a malformed developing fetus (homunculus).

Monodermal teratomas consist of exclusively endodermal or ectodermal tissue types. Struma ovarii is the most common monodermal teratoma of the endoderm. The tumor is seen mainly in postmenopausal patients and may be hormonally active. It has a solid or cystic, greenish brown cut surface. Microscopically, the tumor consists of normal or nodular hyperplastic thyroid tissue (Fig. 11.2). Carcinoids are the second common monodermal teratoma although frequently admixed with other teratomatous components. A third of carcinoids are associated with clinical carcinoid syndromes. Four histological types have been described: insular (the most common, Fig. 11.3), trebecular, strumal carcinoid (mixed carcinoid tumor and struma ovarii), and mucinous carcinoid (carcinoid tumor with goblet cell differentiation). Mucinous carcinoid can be well differentiated (without cytological atypia), atypical (with mild to moderate cytological atypia) or carcinomatous. Monodermal teratoma of the ectoderm includes epidermoid cyst (cystic tumor lined by

D. Chhieng and P. Hui (eds.), *Cytology and Surgical Pathology of Gynecologic Neoplasms*,
Current Clinical Pathology, DOI 10.1007/978-1-60761-164-6_11,
© Springer Science+Business Media, LLC 2011

**Table 11.1** Classification of germ cell tumors of the ovary

| Major heading | Subheading | Variant | Variant | Variant | Variant | Variant | Variant |
|---|---|---|---|---|---|---|---|
| Teratoma | Mature | Solid | Cystic | Fetiform | | | |
| | Monodermal | Struma ovarii | Carcinoid tumor | Strumal carcinoid | Mucinous carcinoid | Epidermoid cyst | Neuroectodermal tumor |
| | Immature | | | | | | |
| Dysgerminoma | Conventional | With trophoblastic differentiation | | | | | |
| Yolk sac tumor | Conventional | Intestinal | Endometrioid | Hepatoid | Polyvesicular viteline | | |
| Embryonal carcinoma | | | | | | | |
| Polyembryoma | | | | | | | |
| Choriocarcinoma | | | | | | | |
| Mixed germ cell tumors | | | | | | | |

**Fig. 11.1** Mature cystic teratoma. Note the ectodermal skin with its appendages and ectodermal neuronal tissues (glia, cerebellum, and choroid plexus) (H.E. ×20)

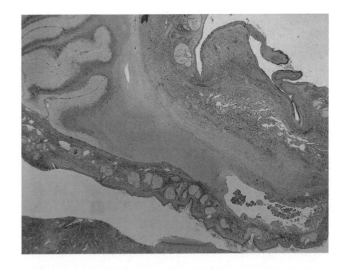

**Fig. 11.2** Strumal ovarii (H.E. ×40)

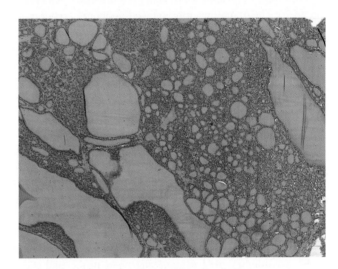

**Fig. 11.3** Carcinoid tumor. Note the insular growth pattern in this case of primary ovarian carcinoid (H.E. ×200)

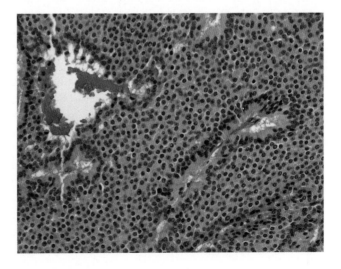

mature squamous epithelium and filled with large amount keratin debris) and neuroectodermal tumors (ependymoma, neuroblastoma, medulloblastoma, PNET, and glioblastoma multiforme).

Malignant tumors may arise from a mature teratoma. Squamous cell carcinoma is the most common. Melanoma and various adenocarcinomas may occur in a mature cystic teratoma. Malignant transformation of a struma ovarii may lead to papillary or follicular thyroid carcinoma.

Immature teratomas are diagnosed when malignant embryonic tissues (particularly the embryonic neuronal tissue) are present, mostly in a background of mature teratoma. They account for 20% ovarian malignancies under the age of 20. The immature embryonic components are predominantly cellular immature glia with scattered neuroepithelial rosettes and tubules (Fig. 11.4a, b). In a poorly differentiated tumor, immature mesodermal (cartilage, bone, skeletal muscle) and endodermal (glands) may be present. The histological grading of the tumor and its metastasis are determined by the percentage of embryonic neuronal components: grade 1 tumor with less than one low power field (4× objective lens) of immature glia in any tumor section; grade 2 tumor with more than one but less than four low power fields of immature glia in any slide; and grade 3 tumor with more than four low power fields of immature glia in any slide. Two-tier grading system has been proposed: low-grade (grade 1) and high grade (combined grades 2 and 3). It is important that the grading is performed on the disorganized embryonic neuronal tissue. Organoid developing fetal tissues should not be counted for the grading, including mitotically active cerebrum, cerebellum, and fetal cartilage. The extent of surgery depends on the patient age, tumor grade, extraovarian spreading, and desire to preserve fertility. High-grade tumors and tumors with peritoneal implants are treated with chemotherapy. In rare cases, implants undergoing chemotherapy-induced maturation may continue to grow (growing teratoma syndrome) and requires additional surgery. Histological grading of the tumor in a child may not be clinically relevant, however.

*Dysgerminoma* is the ovarian counterpart of seminoma of the testis. It is the most common malignant germ cell tumor (50%). Two-thirds of the tumor occur in the second and third decades. The tumor is unilateral in over 90% of the cases and has a size ranging from 1 cm to massive. Grossly, it has a fleshy, whitish gray to pink cut surface. Microscopically, the tumor consists of diffuse proliferation of uniformly large, round immature germ cells that have distinct cell borders, abundant clear cytoplasm and a centrally located nucleus with a prominent central nucleolus (Fig. 11.5a). Rare cases may have focal trophoblastic differentiation in the form of syncytiotrophoblastic giant cells. The stroma consists of thin to thick fibrous septa that are characteristically infiltrated by mature lymphocytes (Fig. 11.5b). Stromal luteinization or prominent granulomatous reaction may be present in some cases. The tumor has an immunohistochemical profile of OCT4+, CD117+, vimentin+, PLAP+, and CD30−.

*Yolk sac tumor* is the second most common malignant germ cell tumor, remarkable for its biosynthesis of alpha-fetal protein. Typically rapidly growing, yolk sac tumor is seen mainly in the second and third decades. The tumor is friable, gray to yellow, frequently hemorrhagic and necrotic. Conventional yolk sac tumor has a reticular to cystic growth pattern. Loosely interconnected tubulocystic spaces are lined by primitive tumor cells (Fig. 11.6a). The tumor cells show marked size and shape variations and have pale to clear glycogen-rich cytoplasm, large hyperchromatic nuclei and prominent nucleoli. Numerous mitotic figures are present. Schiller–Duval bodies are the most characteristic histological findings. These are glomeruloid structures consisting of papillary arrangement of the tumor cells around a central capillary (Fig. 11.6b). Another characteristic finding is the presence intra- and extracellular hyaline bodies (Fig. 11.6c). Typical immunohistochemical

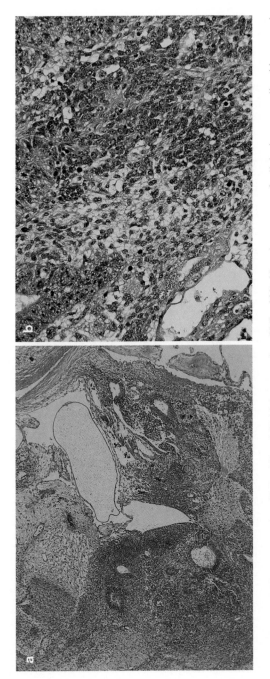

**Fig. 11.4** Immature teratoma. (**a**) Low power view (H.E. ×40) and (**b**) high power view (H.E. ×200). Note the presence of cellular immature glia with scattered neuroepithelial rosettes and tubules. Numerous mitoses are present

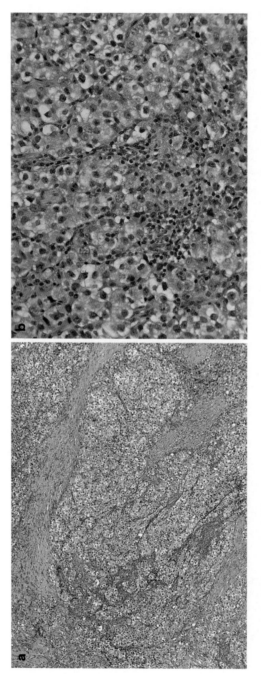

**Fig. 11.5** Dysgerminoma. (**a**) Low power view (H.E. ×40) and (**b**) medium power view (H.E. ×100). Note the diffuse proliferation of uniformly large, round immature germ cells that have distinct cell borders, abundant clear cytoplasm and a centrally located nucleus with a prominent central nucleolus, and the presence of thin to thick fibrous septa infiltrated by mature lymphocytes.

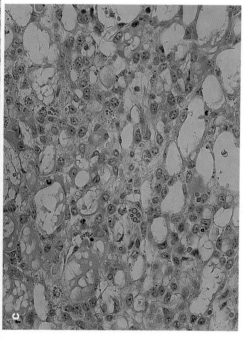

**Fig. 11.6** Yolk sac tumor. (**a**) Note the loosely interconnected tubulocystic spaces are lined by primitive tumor cells (H.E. ×40), (**b**) Schiller–Duval bodies (H.E. ×200), and (**c**) highly atypical cells with marked size and shape variations, clear glycogen-rich cytoplasm, markedly atypical nuclei, intra- and extracellular hyaline globules (H.E. ×200)

profile of the tumor cells includes positivity for AFP, alpha-1 antitrypsin, PLAP and cytokeratin, and negativity for CD117, CK7, EMA, and OCT4. Histological variants of yolk sac tumor include polyvesicular viteline yolk sac tumor (variably sized and shaped cystic spaces lined by flattened tumor cells), hepatoid yolk sac tumor (compact large polygonal cells with abundant eosinophilic cytoplasm and a centrally located nucleus with a large nucleolus) and glandular (intestinal or endometrioid) variants.

*Embryonal carcinoma* is rare and frequently admixed with other types of germ cell tumor. The mean age of the patients is 12 years old. The tumor is a solid growth of large primitive cells with amphophilic cytoplasm. The nuclei are round and vesicular with coarse chromatin and prominent nucleoli. Mitoses are numerous and trophoblastic differentiation in the form of syncytiotrophoblastic giant cells is almost always present. Characteristic immunohistochemical profile includes CD30+, OCT4+, PLAP+, AFP+ and CD117−. Trophoblastic cells are positive for hCG. Near half of the patients present with extraovarian spread at the time of diagnosis.

*Polyembryoma* is a very rare germ cell tumor characterized by the presence of numerous structures simulating normal or malformed early embryos: an embryonic disk, amniotic space, and yolk sac along with surrounding extra-embryonic trophoblasts and mesenchyme. Mixed teratomatous components are usually present. Polyembryoma is a highly aggressive tumor if untreated. Surgery combined with adjuvant chemotherapy is current recommended.

*Nongestational choriocarcinoma* is extremely rare in its pure form but present as a component in 20% of mixed germ cell tumors. Histologically, the tumor is similar to gestational choriocarcinoma. Although the tumor is less responsive to chemotherapy, current cytoreduction surgery combined with chemotherapy results in a cure or long-term remission in some cases.

*Mixed germ cell tumors* account for 10–20% of malignant germ cell tumors. The most common components are dysgerminoma and yolk sac tumor, followed by immature teratoma.

## 11.3 Ovarian Sex Cord-Stromal Tumors

Ovarian sex cord-stromal tumors are derived from ovarian cell types found in the ovarian cortex and hilum with differentiation toward granulose cell, theca cell, gonadal stromal cell, hilar cell, and their related Sertoli and Leydig cell. Thecoma-fibromas are the most common (90%), followed by granulosa cell tumor (7%), Sertoli–Leydig cell tumor (3%), and unclassifiable sex cord-stromal tumors (<0.5%). They are the most common hormone-producing ovarian tumors with clinical manifestation of either hyperestrogenism (granulosa cell tumors) or hyperandrogenism (Sertoli–Leydig cell tumors). Common entities of the ovarian sex cord-stromal tumors are listed in Table 11.2.

### 11.3.1 Granulosa Cell Tumors

Granulosa cell tumors are separated into adult (95%) and juvenile (5%) subtypes. Adult granulose cell tumor is seen in menopausal or postmenopausal women and is the most common functional ovarian tumor associated with clinical hyperestrogenism. The patients present frequently with uterine bleeding, amenorrhea, endometrial hyperplasia, or even endometrioid carcinoma. The tumor is large, cystic, or solid with hemorrhage, and almost always unilateral. Microscopically, the tumor may have various growth patterns: diffuse (Fig. 11.7a), macrofollicular (Fig. 11.7b), microfollicular, insular (Fig. 11.7c), trebecular (Fig. 11.7d), gyriform, pseudopapillary, or sarcomatoid (Fig. 11.7e). The common denominator of all adult granulosa cell tumors is the presence of uniform, round, or oval, haphazardly oriented tumor cells that have pale, angulated nuclei with frequent nuclear grooves (Fig. 11.7f). Call–Exner bodies are rosette-like organization of tumor cells simulating those found developing graafian follicles. They can be numerous in microfollicular granulosa cell tumor (Fig. 11.7g), but may be rare or absent in

**Table 11.2** Histological classifications of ovarian sex cord-stromal tumors

|  | Variant/subtype | Variant/subtype | Variant/subtype | Variant/subtype |
|---|---|---|---|---|
| Granulosa cell tumor | Adult granulosa cell tumor | Juvenile granulosa cell tumor |  |  |
| Thecoma | Thecoma, conventional | Luteinized thecoma |  |  |
| Fibrous tumor | Fibroma | Sclerosing stromal tumor | Signet ring stromal cell tumor | Fibrosarcoma |
| Sertoli-stromal tumor | Sertoli cell tumor | Sertoli–Leydig cell tumor, conventional | Sertoli–Leydig cell tumor, retiform |  |
| Steroid cell tumor | Stromal luetoma | Leydig cell tumor | Hilar cell tumor | Steroid cell tumor, NOS |
| Sex cord tumor with annular tubules |  |  |  |  |
| Gynandroblastoma |  |  |  |  |

others. The mitotic activity is generally low (<3/10 HPF). Frequent mitotic activity, particularly the presence of atypical forms, may be seen in a poorly differentiated granulosa cell tumor, but differential diagnoses should be considered. Rare adult granulosa cell tumors may have scattered bizarre hyperchromatic tumor cells. Reticulin special stain outlines nodules of granulosa cell tumor instead of individual tumor cells seen in thecoma. Characteristic immunohistochemical profile of the tumor cells includes positivity for alpha-inhibin, calretinin, CK8, CK18, S100, and CD99, but negativity for EMA and CK7. Differential diagnoses include undifferentiated carcinoma, small cell carcinoma of hypercalcemic type, thecoma/fibrothecoma, steroid tumor, endometrial stromal sarcoma, endometrioid adenocarcinomas, carcinoid tumor, metastatic breast carcinoma, and metastatic melanoma. Adult granulose cell tumor is notorious for a long-term survival of the patient but eventual tumor recurrences after many years of dormancy.

Juvenile granulosa cell tumor occurs in patients under the age of 30. The tumor causes isosexual pseudoprecocity in prepuberty girls, whereas vaginal bleeding and endometrial hyperplasia in adults. Olier disease (enchondromatosis) and Maffucci syndrome (enchondromatosis and hemangiomatosis) may coexist with the tumor. Similar to the adult type, juvenile granulosa cell tumors are almost always unilateral and large, solid to cystic ovarian masses with hemorrhage. Microscopically, the tumor consists of a diffuse proliferation of granulosa cell in sheets interrupted by varying sizes of follicle-like spaces that may contain basophilic or eosinophilic fluid (Fig. 11.8a). The tumor cells of juvenile granulosa cell tumor are round with eosinophilic or clear luteinized cytoplasm with nongrooved hyperchromatic nuclei (Fig. 11.8b). Luteinized theca cells may form mantles around the follicles. More atypical cells with marked pleomorphism, multinucleation, and mitotic activity are seen in 15% of the cases. Call–Exner bodies are not present in a juvenile granulosa cell tumor. Characteristic immunohistochemical profile of the tumor cells includes positivity for alpha-inhibin, calretinin, and CD99. Differential diagnoses include adult granulosa cell tumor, germ cell tumors, small cell carcinoma of hypercalcemic type, thecoma, clear cell carcinoma, and metastatic melanoma. Only 3% of the stage 1 tumors recur and almost all recurrences happen within 3 years postsurgery.

### 11.3.2 Thecomas and Fibrous Tumors

*Thecomas* are ovarian stromal tumors of lipid containing theca cells, typically seen in a postmenopausal patient and frequently producing

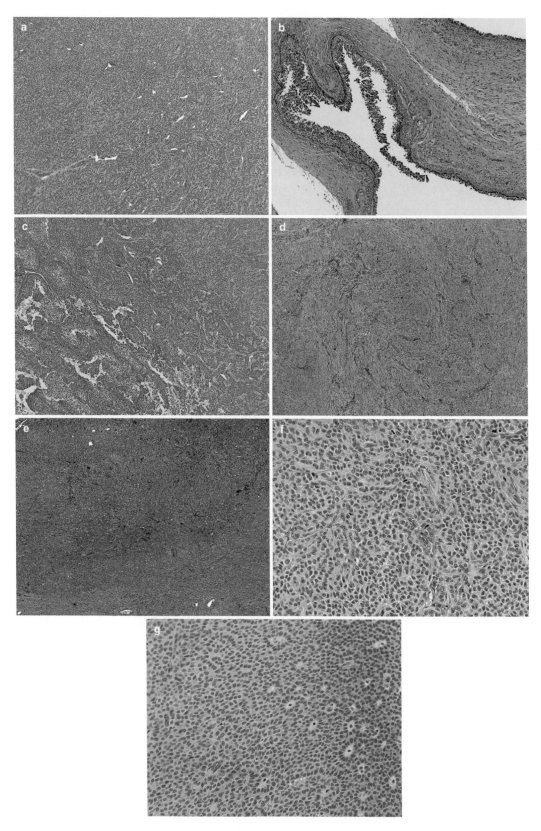

**Fig. 11.7** Adult granulosa cell tumor (AGCT). Note various growth patterns in different tumors: diffuse (**a**), macrofollicular (**b**), insular (**c**), trebecular (**d**), and sarcomatoid (**e**). All tumors have uniform, round or oval, haphazardly oriented tumor cells that have pale, angulated nuclei with frequent nuclear grooves (**f**). Call–Exner bodies are numerous in this microfollicular variant of adult granulosa cell tumor (**g**). All figures are at ×40, except (**f**) and (**g**) (×200)

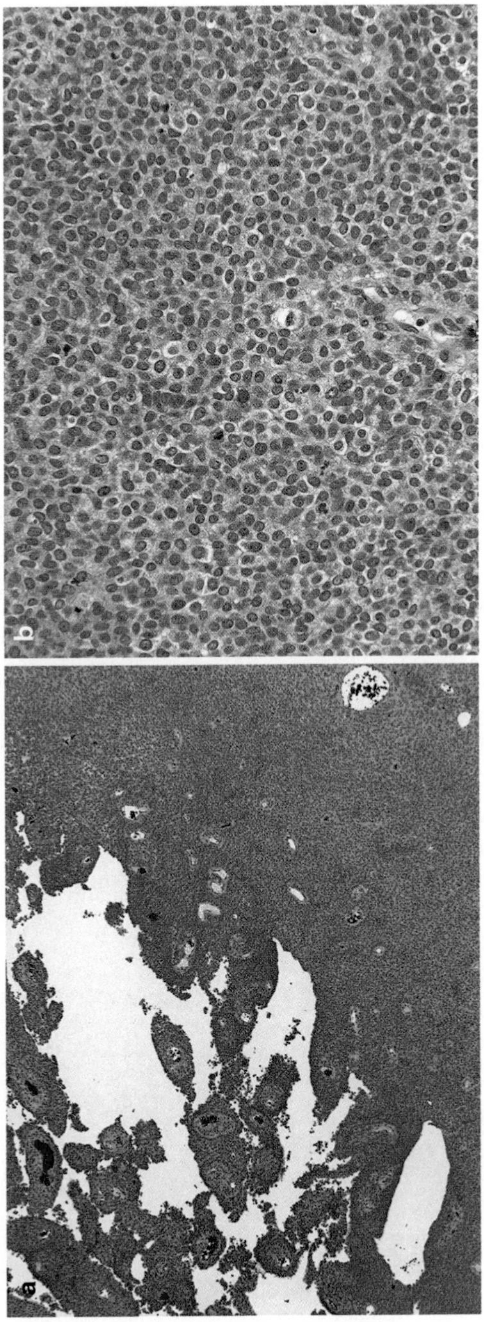

**Fig. 11.8** Juvenile granulosa cell tumor (JGCT). (**a**) Note the diffuse proliferation of granulosa cells in sheets (H.E. ×40). (**b**) The tumor cells are round with eosinophilic or clear luteinized cytoplasm but nongrooved hyperchromatic nuclei (H.E. ×200)

estrogen or androgen. The tumor is solid and yellow. The proliferating cells are round or oval with abundant ill-defined cytoplasm that contains lipid or vacuoles (Fig. 11.9). Sheets of tumor cells are vaguely interspersed by fibrous bands with collagen deposition. No cytological atypia is present, although rare larger bizarre cells of degenerative nature may be present. Fibrothecoma contains significant amount of spindle fibroblastic elements. Reticulin fiber is present around each tumor cell or rarely small groups of tumor cells, in contrast to the absence of reticulin within tumor nests in a granulosa cell tumor.

*Luteinized thecoma* is a fibromatous or thecomatous tumor with the presence of single or small nests of luteinized cells that stand out as large round cells with abundant clear cytoplasm. Rare luteinized thecoma occurs in association with sclerosing peritonitis, a spindle cell proliferation containing numerous lutein cells involving peritoneum.

*Sclerosing stromal tumor* is a benign spindle cell tumor in young adult with a mean age of 27 years. These are solid tumors with yellow edematous cut surface. Lobulated cellular proliferation alternating with paucicellular edematous area is characteristic (Fig. 11.10). The proliferating cells are short spindle, vacuolated lutein cells and fibroblasts with a sclerosing background of collagen deposition and hemangiopericytomatous vasculatures. The tumor cells are immunoreactive to vimentin, alpha-inhibin, calretinin, SMA, and CD34.

*Signet-ring stromal tumor* is a stromal tumor with diffuse presence of vacuolated cells of signet-ring cell appearance in a background of fibroma. This rare tumor is seen in an adult patient, and the main differential diagnosis is Krukenberg tumor.

### 11.3.3 Sertoli-Stromal Cell Tumors

1. *Sertoli cell tumors* are usually nonfunctional tumors in a young woman (mean age of 30). Rare lipid-rich variant may produce estrogen and the oxyphilic type may be associated with Peutz–Jeghers syndrome. The tumor consists of lobules of hollow or solid tubules lined by columnar or cuboidal cells with pale to eosinophilic cytoplasm. Lipid rich tumors have strikingly clear lipid laden cytoplasm. Absence of Leydig cells separates it from a Sertoli–Leydig cell tumor (see below).

2. *Sertoli–Leydig cell tumors* account for less than 0.5% of ovarian tumors with more than two-third diagnosed under the age of 30. They produce androgen leading to clinical virilization in 30–50% of the cases. Almost always unilateral, these tumors are yellow with solid to cystic cut surface. The tumors are subtyped

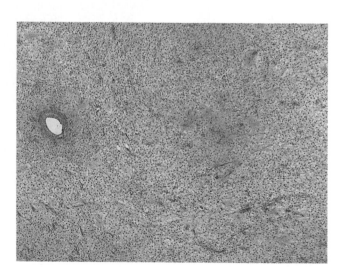

**Fig. 11.9** Thecoma. Note sheets of round or oval tumor cells with abundant ill-defined cytoplasm that contains lipid or vacuolated (H.E. ×40)

**Fig. 11.10** Sclerosing stromal tumor. Note the lobulated cellular proliferation alternating with paucicellular edematous area and hemangiopericytoma-like vasculatures (H.E. ×40)

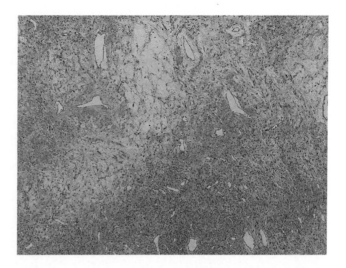

histologically into well differentiated (10%), intermediate-differentiated (50%) and poorly differentiated (35%). Well-differentiated tumors consist of lobules of tubular proliferation of mature Sertoli cells (columnar to cuboidal in shape and containing eosinophilic cytoplasm and small round or angulated nuclei), intimately admixed with single to nest of Leydig cells (Fig. 11.11a). Reinke crystals may be found in Leydig cells but absent in many cases. Intermediately differentiated tumors have lobules or irregular masses of solid sheets, cords, or nests of immature Sertoli cells, separated by fibrous bands (Fig. 11.11b). Subtle abortive tubular formations and rare hollow tubules may be appreciated. Mitoses are commonly present. Leydig cell aggregates are present at the periphery of the lobules (Fig. 11.11c). Poorly differentiated tumors are solid and sarcomatoid with immature, spindled Sertoli cells arranged in only vague trabecular pattern (Fig. 11.11d). There are numerous mitotic figures. Leydig cell may be lacking or difficult to be found. Sertoli–Leydig cell tumor with heterologous elements is seen in one-fifth of the cases, such as mature to immature mucinous glands, cartilage, and muscle.

Retiform Sertoli–Leydig cell tumor is seen in patients of younger age (mean age of 15 years). The tumor has growth patterns resembling the rete testis but frequently admixed with conventional Sertoli–Leydig cell tumor of intermediate to poor differentiation. The tumor may be cystic grossly. Histologically, it consists of elongated, slit-like tubules, or papillae of various calibers (Fig. 11.11e). Solid tubules or nest of immature Sertoli cells are easily found.

Sertoli–Leydig cell tumors have an immunohistochemical profile with cells positive for vimentin, cytokeratin, alpha-inhibin, calretinin, PR, and androgen receptor. Differential diagnoses are broad, including ovarian epithelial tumors (endometrioid and serous carcinoma), Krukenberg tumor, trabecular carcinoid tumor, struma ovarii, ependymoma, teratoma, and yolk sac tumor. All clinically malignant Sertoli–Leydig cells tumor are of poorly differentiated ones and those with mesenchymal heterologous components. Retiform tumor appears to be more aggressive in general although inconclusive. Intraabdominal spread without distant metastasis is typical.

### 11.3.4  Steroid Cell Tumors

Steroid cell tumors are rare hormone-secretion tumors with cells resembling lutein cells, Leydig cell, or adrenal cortical cells. All types of steroid cell tumors express alpha-inhibin and may

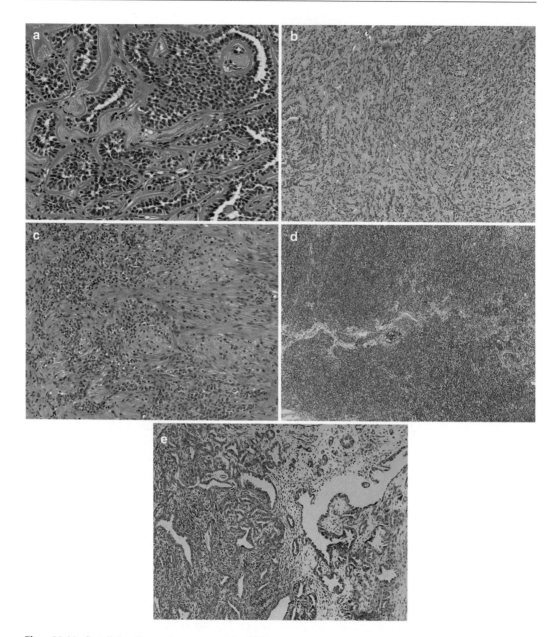

**Fig. 11.11** Sertoli–Leydig cell tumor. (**a**) Well-differentiated tumors consist of lobules of tubular proliferation of mature Sertoli cells (H.E. ×200). (**b**) Intermediately differentiated tumors have lobules or irregular masses of solid sheets, cords or nests of immature Sertoli cells, separated by fibrous bands (H.E. ×100). (**c**) Leydig cell aggregates are present at the periphery of the lobules (H.E. ×100). (**d**) Poorly differentiated tumors are solid and sarcomatoid with immature, spindled Sertoli cells arranged in only vague trabecular pattern (H.E. ×40). (**e**) Rete form Sertoli–Leydig cell tumor has growth patterns resembling the rete testis (H.E. ×100)

contain minor foci of pleomorphic cells of degenerative nature.

1. *Pregnancy luteoma* is a tumor-like condition, frequently seen as an incidental finding during the cesarean section or tubal ligation procedures. The tumor is bilateral in one-third of the cases. It is average of 7.0 cm in size and is red to yellow solid. Histologically, it is well demarcated from the ovarian

stroma and consists of luteinized steroid cells (Fig. 11.12). Mitotic activity may be abundant. Dystrophic calcification may be present.

2. *Stromal luteomas* are benign, unilateral small (<3 cm) tumors arising from the ovarian stroma and associated with stromal hyperthecosis in a postmenopausal patient. The patients commonly present with hyperestrinism (60%) or masculinization (20%). The tumor consists of nodular growth of lipid-depleted lutein cells in nest or diffuses arrangements, surrounded by ovarian stroma, which may be hyalinized.

3. *Leydig cell tumors* are mostly found within the hilum of the ovary (hilus cell tumor). The patients typically present with virilization (80%). The tumor is unilateral, reddish-brown nodule consisting of Leydig cells with abundant eosinophilic cytoplasm and identifiable Reinke crystals (Fig. 11.13). Hilar cell hyperplasia is frequently present. Leydig cell tumors are benign.

4. *Steroid cell tumors, not otherwise specified* account for 60% of steroid cell tumors. The patients are generally younger with a mean age of 43 years. These unilateral tumors are larger (8.0 cm in average) and have a yellow-brown

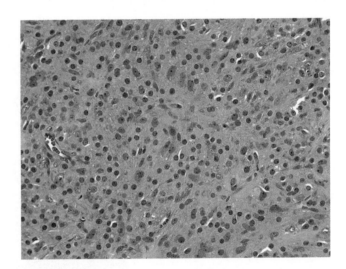

**Fig. 11.12** Pregnancy luteoma (H.E. ×200)

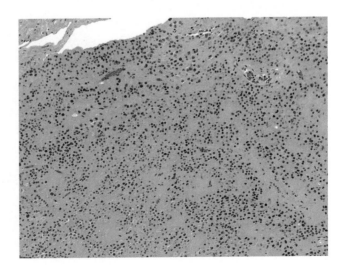

**Fig. 11.13** Leydig cell tumor (H.E. ×100)

cut surface. Microscopically, the tumor consists of diffuse proliferation of large polygonal or round cell with abundant eosinophilic or lipid-rich cytoplasm (Fig. 11.14) and centrally located small nuclei. One-third of the tumors are clinically malignant. Large tumor size (>7 cm), two or more mitosis/10 HPF, necrosis, hemorrhage, and significant nuclear atypia are features associated with clinical malignancy.

*Sex cord tumor with annular tubules (SCTAT)* is a rare but histologically distinct tumor involving young patients in their 20s or 30s. Peutz–Jeghers syndrome is present in one-third of the cases and associated with bilateral tumors. The tumors are unilateral and produce estrogen when not associated with Peutz–Jeghers syndrome,

however. Microscopically, the tumor consists of distinct simple to complex ring-shaped tubular structures containing cribriform or punched-out acellular hyalinized spaces. Palisading of tumor cells around the periphery of the nests is characteristic. Calcification or psammoma bodies are frequently present. Tumors associated with Peutz–Jeghers syndrome are almost always benign, whereas those without are clinically malignant in 20% of the cases.

*Gonadoblastoma* is a tumor arising from dysgenetic gonads of 46XY genotype. The tumor is composed of immature germ cells (dysgerminoma, yolk sac tumor or others) and sex cord-stromal cells (granulosa cell tumor or Sertoli cell tumors). Leydig cells are present in the stroma (Fig. 11.15).

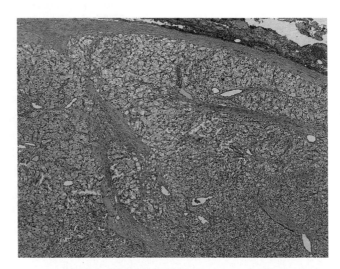

**Fig. 11.14** Steroid cell tumor, not otherwise specified. Note the diffuse proliferation of large polygonal or round cell with abundant eosinophilic or lipid-rich cytoplasm (H.E. ×40)

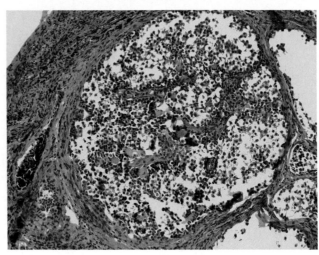

**Fig. 11.15** Gonadoblastoma (H.E. ×100)

*Gynandroblastomas* are very rare tumors of young adult with histological differentiations toward both granulosa-stromal and Sertoli-stromal cells. They are almost always benign clinically.

as primary ovarian masses, including leiomyoma, leiomyosarcoma, hemangioma, angiosarcoma, adenomatoid tumor, paraganglioma, and myxoma. Primary ovarian ependymoma is a rare tumor with histological similarity to that of the CNS primary (Fig. 11.18).

## 11.4  Miscellaneous Primary Ovarian Tumors

Primary lymphomas: diffuse large B cell lymphoma (Fig. 11.16) and Burkitt's lymphoma (Fig. 11.17) are two most common primary lymphomas of the ovary. Varieties of soft tissue tumors rarely occur

## 11.5  Cytology

### 11.5.1  Mature Cystic Teratomas

The most common germ tumor involving the ovary is mature cystic teratoma. Aspirates from

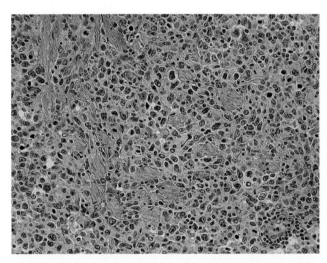

**Fig. 11.16**  Diffuse large B cell lymphoma (H.E. ×200)

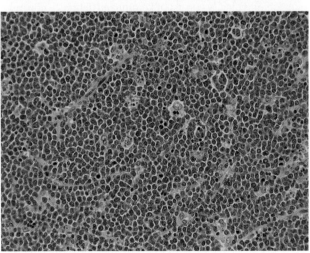

**Fig. 11.17**  Burkett's lymphoma (H.E. ×200)

**Fig. 11.18** Eppendymoma
(H.E. ×100)

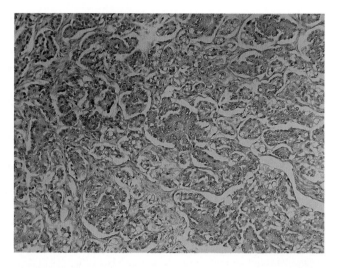

**Fig. 11.19** Mature Cystic
Teratomas. Tissue fragment
consisting of keratinized debris,
anucleated squames, and
squamous cells are noted (cell
block preparation, H.E. ×100)

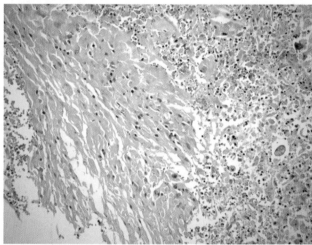

such tumor typically consist of keratinized debris, squamous cells, and other amorphous debris (Fig. 11.19). Other cellular components that may be present include sebaceous cells, adipose tissue, intestinal, and respiratory type epithelium, cartilage, and hair strands.

chromatin, and prominent nucleoli. Small mature lymphocytes are usually present (Fig. 11.20). Trigoid background, best appreciated with Diff-Quik stain, are noted in less than half of the cases.

## 11.5.2 Dysgerminoma

Dysgerminoma may rarely undergo cystic changes. Cytologically, it resembles its testicular counterpart and is characterized by large neoplastic cells with round nuclei, vesicular

## 11.5.3 Other Germ Cell Tumors

Nonseminomatous germ cell tumors include embryonal carcinoma, yolk sac tumor, and choriocarcinoma. The aspirates of these tumors often demonstrate cohesive groups of pleomorphic

**Fig. 11.20** Dysgerminoma.
Predominantly discohesive large
cells with vesicular nuclei and
prominent nucleoli. Small, round
lymphocytes are noted in the
background (ThinPrep,
Papanicolaou, ×400)

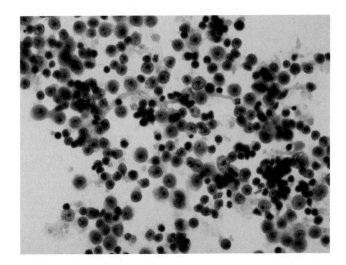

epithelioid cells with prominent nucleoli. The
cytoplasm is usually scant with indistinct cell
borders, resulting in a syncytial growth pattern.
In addition, the neoplastic cells can also demonstrate a papillary and/or glandular arrangement.
Necrosis is frequently noted, resulting in a cystic
appearance.

### 11.5.4 Granulosa Cell Tumors

The majority of the sex cord-stromal tumors are
solid tumors with the exception of granulose cell
tumors, which are partly solid and partly cystic.

Aspirates are cellular and consist of relatively uniform cells singly or in loosely cohesive clusters.
Rosettes formation may be noted. The tumor cells
are small with scant cytoplasm, oval nuclei with
nuclear grooves and distinct nucleoli.

## Suggested Reading

Clement PB, Young RH. Atlas of Gynecologic Surgical
    Pathology. Saunders Publisher, Philadelphia, PA, 2008.
Kurman R. Blaustein's Pathology of the Female Genital
    Tract. 5th Edition. Springer, Berlin, 2002.
Prat J. Pathology of the Ovary. Saunders Publisher,
    Philadelphia, PA, 2004.

# Chapter 12
# Tumors of Peritoneum

**Keywords** Peritoneum • Mesothelioms • Ascites • Pelvic washing • Immunohistochemistry

## 12.1 General Classification of Tumors of Peritoneum

Primary peritoneal tumors and tumor-like conditions of secondary mullerian system include various endometrioid, serous, and mucinous lesions. Endometriosis is the most common tumor-like condition resulting in a significant morbidity in women of reproductive years of age. In addition, preneoplastic hyperplasia and carcinomas (clear cell and endometrioid carcinomas) may arise from endometriosis. Primary peritoneal serous carcinoma is a frequent differential diagnosis from that of the ovarian primary. Diffuse involvement of surfaces of various abdominal organs and minimal (<5 mm in size) ovarian parenchymal involvement are diagnostic criteria for a peritoneal serous carcinoma. Various serous and mucinous cytadenomas and borderline tumors may present as extraovarian primaries. Metastatic carcinomas are the most common tumors involving the peritoneum. Gestational trophoblastic tumors primarily involving the peritoneum are extremely rare, including gestational choriocarcinoma and intermediate trophoblastic tumor (PSTT and ETT, see Chap. 8).

## 12.2 Mesotheliomas

Mesotheliomas of the peritoneum may be classified into benign (adenomatoid tumor, benign multicystic mesothelioma, well-differentiated papillary mesothelioma) and malignant (malignant mesothelioma and intraabdominal desmoplastic small round cell tumor).

*Adenomatoid tumors* generally involve the uterus and fallopian tube, and only rarely arise from the peritoneal mesothelium.

*Multicystic mesothelioma* or mesothelial cyst is usually an incidental finding during a laparotomy. The lesion consists of multilocular cysts containing clear fluid and lined by simple benign mesothelium (Fig. 12.1). The lesion is benign.

*Well-differentiated papillary mesotheliomas* are solitary or multiple papillary proliferations of mesothelial cells. The lesions are usually small (<2 cm) and involve pelvic peritoneum and omentum. The papillae are covered by monolayer of cuboidal to flattened mature mesothelial cells (Fig. 12.2). The stroma may be edematous to fibrous. Solitary lesions are benign. When multiple lesions are present, each lesion should be carefully sampled to rule out concurrent invasive malignant mesothelioma.

*Malignant mesotheliomas* of the peritoneum in female are not associated with occupational exposure to asbestos. The gross and microscopic features are similar to those involving the pleura.

D. Chhieng and P. Hui (eds.), *Cytology and Surgical Pathology of Gynecologic Neoplasms*, Current Clinical Pathology, DOI 10.1007/978-1-60761-164-6_12, © Springer Science+Business Media, LLC 2011

**Fig. 12.1** Multicystic
mesothelioma. Note the
multilocular cysts containing
clear fluid and lined by simple
benign mesothelium (H&E, ×20)

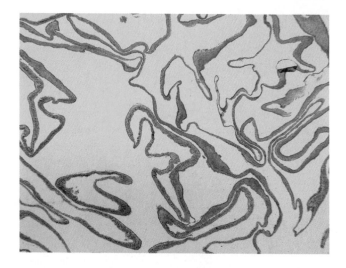

**Fig. 12.2** Well-differentiated
papillary mesothelioma. Note the
papillary proliferation and
single layer of cuboidal to
flattened mature mesothelial cells
(H&E, ×40)

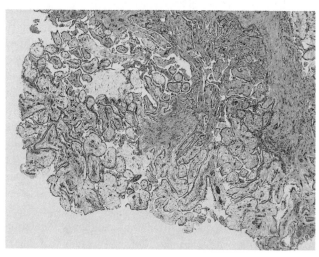

Most tumors are epithelial type with tubulopapillary or papillary growth patterns (Fig. 12.3a, b). Solid, sarcomatoid, biphasic, or deciduoid variants are encountered in rare cases. The major differential diagnosis is mullerian serous carcinoma. Tubulopapillary growth, relatively uniform polygonal tumor cells, mild to moderate nuclear atypia, uncommon mitotic figures and immunohistochemical positivity for caldesmon and calretinin but ER and Ber-EP4 are features strongly favor mesothelioma over serous carcinoma.

*Intraabdominal desmoplastic small round-cell tumor* is of uncertain histogenesis although a mesothelial origin has been proposed. This is generally a pediatric tumor involving adolescents and young adults of both genders. The tumor consists of multinodular firm masses involving peritoneal surface with invasion of the underlying organs. Microscopically, the tumor is characterized by solid growth of epithelioid cells in sheet or nest that are separated by prominent desmoplastic fibrous component (Fig. 12.4a, b). The tumor cells are uniform small to medium size with indistinct cell borders and little cytoplasm. The nuclei are typically round to oval and hyperchromatic with inconspicuous nucleoli. Numerous mitoses are present. The tumor cells are characteristically positive for cytokeratin, NSE, desmin, WT-1, and vimentin. Staining of CD99, MOC-31, Ber-EP-4, and neuroendocrine markers may also be positive in some cases. Molecular demonstration of $t(11;22)$ translocation or its associated chimeric transcript between EWS and WT genes is diagnostic. This is a

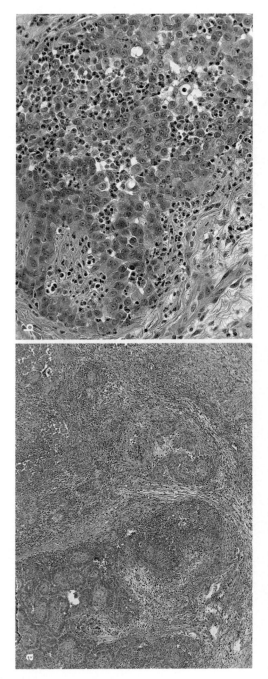

**Fig. 12.3** Malignant mesothelioma. This epithelial type mesothelioma consists of invasive tubulopapillary to papillary growth of uniform polygonal tumor cells with mild to moderate nuclear atypia. (**a**) Low power view (H&E, ×40) and (**b**) high power view (H&E, ×200)

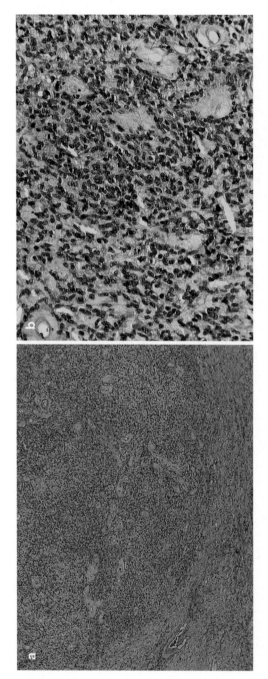

**Fig. 12.4** Desmoplastic small round cell tumor. Note the solid growth of epithelioid cells in sheet or nest that are sharply separated by prominent desmoplastic fibrous component (**a**) (H&E, ×40). The tumor cells are uniform, small to medium sized with indistinct cell borders and little cytoplasm. The nuclei are typically round to oval and hyperchromatic with inconspicuous nucleoli (**b**) (H&E, ×200).

highly aggressive tumor with a mortality over 90% regardless of surgery and/or chemotherapy at current time.

## 12.3 Other Mesenchymal Tumors

Diffuse Intraabdominal leiomyomatosis is rare smooth muscle proliferation characterized by the presence of several to numerous subserosal nodules of leiomyomas of <1 cm in size (see Chap. 7). Other mesenchymal tumors include solitary fibrous tumor, inflammatory myofibroblastic tumor, calcifying fibrous tumor, and various sarcomas.

## 12.4 Cytology

Peritoneal cytology plays an important role in the diagnosis and staging of many abdominal and gynecologic neoplasms. For example, ascites may be the initial presentation of these neoplasms or the first sign of disease recurrence and diagnosis can be confirmed by cytologic examination of the peritoneal fluids. For patients with gynecologic neoplasms, peritoneal washing cytology has been utilized in the initial resection as well as the second look laparotomies to provide valuable information that can impact

prognosis and therapeutic decision, particularly in the absence of gross evidence of peritoneal involvement. Brushings and/or scraping from the surfaces of the liver and diaphragm can also been used to determine if there is any disease extension beyond the pelvic. To minimize iatrogenic contamination, peritoneal washing should be performed as an initial step of the laparotomy before any exploration.

### 12.4.1 Cytology of Benign and Nonneoplastic Conditions

Normal mesothelial cells do not exfoliate. Therefore, any exfoliated mesothelial cells present are a response to the pathologic process causing the ascites. These reactive mesothelial cells can appear singly or in groups of variable sizes. The latter can be three-dimensional clusters, papillae, cell-in-cell, and even single filing. The cellular clusters often demonstrate lobulated, knobby borders. A characteristic feature is the presence of clear space, or window between adjacent cells due to the presence of long microvilli on the surface of the cells (Figs. 12.5 and 12.6). Another characteristic feature is that cytoplasm is dense in the central area (due to perinuclear accumulation of filaments) and pale in the periphery, resulting in

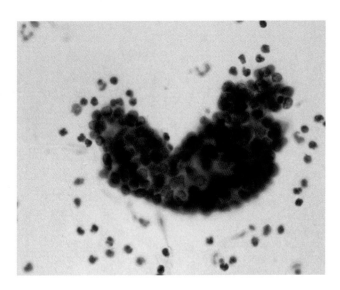

**Fig. 12.5** Reactive mesothelial cells. A three-dimensional papillary group of reactive mesothelial cells (ThinPrep, Papanicolaou, ×400)

two-tone staining. Blunt cytoplasmic processes or projections as well as cytoplasmic vacuoles may be noted. The nuclei are usually central or slightly eccentrically located. Nucleoli range from inconspicuous to prominent. Bi- and multinucleation are common. Mitotic figures may be present but are not indicative of malignancy. Reactive mesothelial cells can demonstrate a wide range of morphologic appearance.

Another cellular component is histiocytes which tend to have indistinct cytoplasmic borders and sometimes phagocytic vacuoles (Fig. 12.7). They do not form papillae and three-dimensional cohesive groups. Histiocytes may be difficult to

distinguish from reactive mesothelial cells. Cells from lung, liver, muscle, cartilage, skin, and appendages, and fat can be seen from time to time in fluid as they are "picked up" by the needle during paracentesis.

For peritoneal washing, the mesothelial cells are often stripped from the underlying connective tissue and therefore, appear as two-dimensional, honey-comb like, flat sheets. The latter can be folded or compressed (Fig. 12.8). The nuclei are round to oval and centrally located with fine granular chromatin and usually a small, distinct nucleolus. Bi-lobulation, nuclear grooves, and multinucleation may be

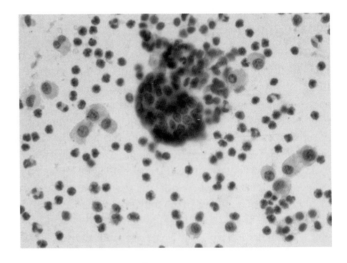

**Fig. 12.6** Reactive mesothelial cells. Papillary group of mesothelial cells with nuclear enlargement and distinct nucleoli (ThinPrep, Papanicolaou, ×400)

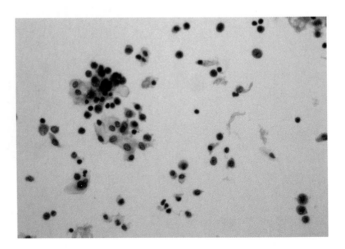

**Fig. 12.7** Histiocytes. Predominantly discohesive epithelioid cells with slightly eccentric nuclei and abundant foamy cytoplasm (ThinPrep, Papanicolaou, ×400)

**Fig. 12.8** Pelvic washing. Monolayered sheet of mesothelial cells with round to oval to kidney shaped nuclei, abundant nondescript cytoplasm, and well-defined cytoplasmic borders (ThinPrep, Papanicolaou, ×400)

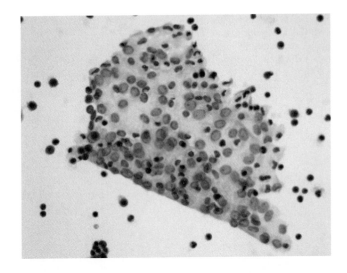

**Fig. 12.9** Endosalpingiosis. Small clusters of cuboidal cells with scant cytoplasm and bland appearing nuclei. Ciliated cytoplasm is noted (see *circle*) (ThinPrep, Papanicolaou, ×400)

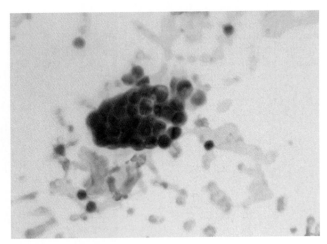

seen. The cytoplasm is thin and polygonal in shape.

### 12.4.1.1 Endosalpingiosis

It is characterized by the presence of scattered small clusters and papillary groups of cuboidal and low columnar cells with scant cytoplasm and round to oval and bland nuclei (Fig. 12.9). A definitive diagnosis relies on the identification of cilia. The differential diagnosis includes serous neoplasia especially when there are many and/or large cell clusters with features suggesting endosalpingiosis.

### 12.4.1.2 Collagen Balls

They appear round to oval nodules of collagen, which appears metachromatic with Diff-Quik stain and pale blue with Papanicolaou stain, surrounded by flattened mesothelial cells (Fig. 12.10). The finding of collagen balls has no clinical significance.

### 12.4.2 Psammoma Bodies

Psammoma bodies are round structures that are composed on concentric laminated circles of calcification (Figs. 12.11 and 12.12). Psammoma

**Fig. 12.10** Collagen balls.
Ova nodules of blue extracellular
matrix surrounded by mesothelial
cells (ThinPrep, Papanicolaou,
×400)

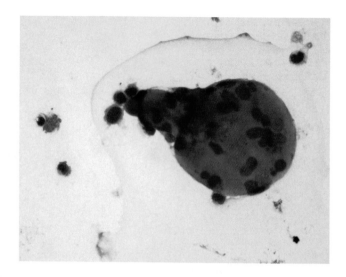

**Fig. 12.11** Psammoma bodies.
Calcified body with concentric
laminations and associated
metastatic ovarian carcinoma
(cell block, H&E, ×200)

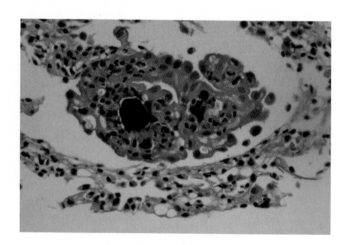

**Fig. 12.12** Psammoma bodies.
Calcified body with concentric
laminations and associated
reactive mesothelial cells
(ThinPrep, Papanicolaou, ×400)

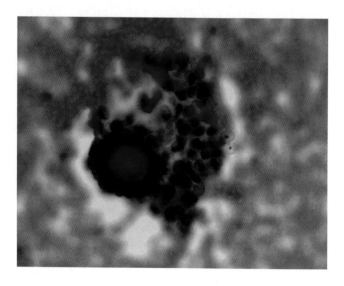

bodies can be observed in 16% of peritoneum fluid specimens. About 55% of cases with psammoma bodies are associated with malignant neoplasms. The remaining 45% of cases are associated with various benign conditions, including ovariancystadenoma/cystadenofibroma, papillary mesothelial hyperplasia, endosalpingiosis, and endometriosis.

## 12.4.3 Neoplastic Conditions

### 12.4.3.1 Metastatic Adenocarcinoma

The key to diagnose a metastatic adenocarcinoma in fluid specimens is the finding of foreign cells with malignant features (Fig. 12.13). At low magnification, tumor cells form large aggregates, cell balls, papillae, and acini. Cell balls, often multiple, are round cellular aggregates with smooth, community borders. "Cannonballs" refer to the presence of large cell balls and are diagnostic of a metastatic malignancy. Acini are three-dimensional clusters with hollow center. Papillae are three-dimensional clusters that are longer in one dimension than in the others. Neoplastic cells can also arrange in chains or "Indian file." Single cells are frequent. Rarely, signet ring cells with large cells may be present. The background is usually nonspecific.

Individual malignant cells appear round to oval with nuclear enlargement, high N/C ratio,

irregular nuclear membranes, and prominent nucleoli (Fig. 12.14). However, hyperchormasia may not be obvious. The cell borders are poorly defined and the cytoplasm is often basophilic and may contain vacuoles. Giant cells and multinucleated cells can be seen.

Mesothelial cells, both reactive and malignant, can mimic metastatic adenocarcinoma and therefore, can result in both false positive and negative diagnoses. Table 12.1 summarizes the differential features for adenocarcinoma and mesothelial cells in fluids.

### 12.4.3.2 Borderline Serous Ovarian Tumors

It is characterized by the presence of branching papillary groups with smooth border. Individual cells demonstrate mild to moderate cytologic atypia with high N:C ratio, slightly irregular nuclear membranes, and inconspicuous nucleoli (Figs. 12.15 and 12.16). Despite the cytologic atypia, the nuclei often appear monomorphic. Cytoplasm is scant with infrequent vacuolation. Single cells are usually rare and psammoma bodies can be present.

Differential diagnosis includes mesothelial hyperplasia, endosalpingosis, and well-differentiated serous carcinoma. The papillary groups in mesothelial hyperplasia are less likely to demonstrate branching. The finding of ciliated

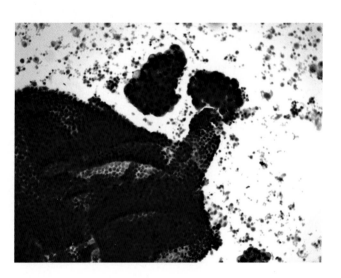

**Fig. 12.13** Metastatic ovarian carcinoma. Two types of cells are present. Reactive mesothelial cells arranged in two-dimensional sheets and metastatic ovarian carcinoma in three-dimensional clusters (ThinPrep, Papanicolaou, ×100)

cells favors endosalpingiosis. The presence of conspicuous number of single atypical cells suggests a carcinoma.

### 12.4.3.3  Pseudomyxoma Peritonei

It is referred to the presence of abundant amount of mucinous material in the peritoneal cavity in association with a low-grade mucin-producing tumor. The latter is often originated from ovary, appendix, or both. Rarely, other gastrointestinal, pancreatic, and uterine neoplasms may also be the sources. Cytologically, the specimen is composed of thick mucus which is difficult to smear (Fig. 12.17). The tumor cells are often sparse and consist of cohesive sheets and strips of bland-appearing tall columnar cells with mucin vacuoles, resembling endocervical epithelium.

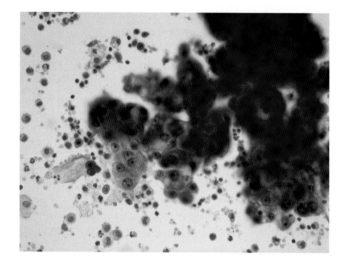

**Fig. 12.14** Metastatic ovarian carcinoma. Individual cells demonstrate moderate amount of cytoplasm with infrequent vacuolation. Nuclei are markedly enlarged with vesicular chromatin and prominent macronucleoli (ThinPrep, Papanicolaou, ×400)

**Table 12.1** Differential diagnosis of adenocarcinomas and mesothelial cells in fluid

| Cytologic features | Mesothelial cells | Adenocarcinoma |
|---|---|---|
| *Presentation* | No foreign cells | Foreign cells with malignant features |
| *Cell arrangement* | | |
| Cell balls | Lobulated, knobby borders | Smooth, community borders |
| Acinar pattern | Absent (intercellular window mistaken as lumen) | Present |
| Cell-in-cell pattern | Present | Absent |
| Intercellular window | Present | Absent |
| Signet ring cells | Rare | Sometimes |
| *Cytoplasm* | | |
| Borders | Well defined | Variable |
| Texture | Dense center, with pale periphery | Homogeneous |
| Staining | Two tone | Uniform |
| Cytoplasmic blebs | Present | Absent |
| *Nuclei* | | |
| Location | Central or paracentral | Eccentric |
| Bi- and multinucleation | Common | Rare |
| N/C ratio | Variable | Moderate to markedly increase |

**Fig. 12.15** Serous borderline tumor. Papillary groups of mildly atypical glandular cells (cytospin, Diff-Quik, ×200)

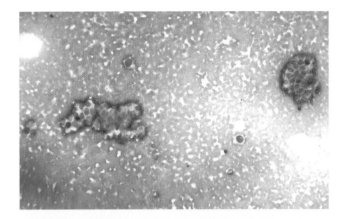

**Fig. 12.16** Serous borderline tumor. Papillary groups of mildly atypical glandular cells associated with psammoma bodies (cell block preparation, H&E, ×200)

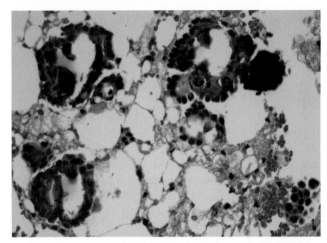

**Fig. 12.17** Pseudomyxoma peritonei. Scattered histiocytes in a background of abundant mucin. No epithelial cells are noted in this example (direct smear, Papanicolaou, ×400)

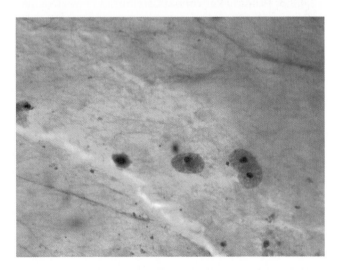

### 12.4.3.4 Primary Malignant Mesothelioma

To correctly diagnose mesothelioma on cytology, one needs to recognize its mesothelial origin and its malignant nature. Table 12.2 summarizes the differential diagnosis between reactive mesothelial cells and mesothelioma. Unfortunately, there is much overlap in the morphology between

**Table 12.2** Differential diagnosis between reactive mesothelial cells and mesothelioma in cytology

| Cytologic features | Reactive mesothelial cells | Mesothelioma |
|---|---|---|
| *Cellularity* | Variable | Highly cellular |
| *Cell arrangement* | | |
| Flat, monolayered sheets | Frequent | Infrequent |
| Three-dimensional cell groups | Fewer, smaller, and flatter | Abundant, large, and more complex |
| Papillae | Less frequent | More frequent |
| *Cells* | | |
| Size | | Larger and more variable |
| Spindle-shaped cells | Absent | Sometimes |
| Giant and multinucleated cells | Rare | Frequent |
| Nuclear membrane | Smooth | Irregular |
| Macronucleoli | Absent | Present |
| *Immunophenotyping* | | |
| EMA (membranous) | 16% | 75% |
| Desmin (cytoplasmic) | 84% | 22% |
| p53 (nuclear) | 8% (weak and few) | 57% |
| *Aneuploidy* | 0% | 53% |

mesothelioma and reactive mesothelial cells (Fig. 12.18). One important clue in diagnosing mesothelioma is the presence of "more and bigger cells in more and bigger clusters" at low power magnification. In some instances, the differences between the two entities can be quite subtle.

### 12.4.3.5 Primary Peritoneal Carcinoma

Cytologically, primary peritoneal carcinoma is indistinguishable from metastatic ovarian serous carcinoma.

### 12.4.3.6 Role of Peritoneal Washing Cytology in Gynecologic Malignancies

Peritoneal washing is recommended for patients who undergo laparotomy for gynecologic neoplasm. The purpose is to detect any occult extraovarian or uterine spread of disease in patients with locally confined tumor. Patients with a negative peritoneal washing are more likely to have a better prognosis than patients with a positive peritoneal washing. In most instances, a positive peritoneal washing is often associated with other poor prognostic findings, such as nodal metastasis

or extrauterine involvement, and therefore does not have independent prognostic value. However, a positive peritoneal washing can negate other favorable prognostic factors, which can result in the need for additional radiation or chemotherapy. Therefore, peritoneal washing status is incorporated in the FIGO staging protocol for both ovarian and endometrial carcinoma.

For patients with ovarian carcinoma, a positive peritoneal washing will raise the stage from FIGO Stage IA or 1B to Stage IC. For patients with endometrial carcinoma, the incidence of positive washing ranges from 7 to 20% for all stages. Patients with well-differentiated endometrial carcinomas with only minimal or superficial myometrial invasion are rarely associated with positive peritoneal washing. Nonetheless, according to the current staging protocol, a positive peritoneal cytology in women with disease confined to the uterus will result in upstaging from Stage I or II to III. However, the data regarding the prognostic value of positive peritoneal cytology in women with Stage I and II endometrial carcinoma has been conflicting.

Seven to twenty-one percent of patients with cervical carcinoma have positive peritoneal washing and is almost always associated with other poor prognostic factors. Patients with adenocarcinomas are more likely to have positive

**Fig. 12.18** Malignant Mesothelioma, well differentiated. Small papillary groups of mesothelial cells with moderate nuclear enlargement and distinct nucleoli. The cytology morphology overlaps with that of reactive mesothelial cells. Subsequent biopsy reveals invasion of the underlying stroma by neoplastic mesothelial cells (ThinPrep, Papanicolaou, ×400)

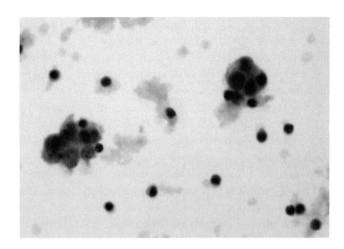

peritoneal washing than those with squamous cell carcinomas.

## 12.4.4 Ancillary Studies

### 12.4.4.1 Mesothelial Cells Versus Adenocarcinoma

Various ancillary studies are often used to help in the distinction between mesothelial cells and adenocarcinomas. Demonstration of neutral mucin production by cytochemistry, particularly mucicarmine, differentiates adenocarcinoma from mesothelial cells. However, cytochemical stains are relatively insensitive. In addition, up to 2–5% of the well-moderately differentiated mesotheliomas are mucicarmine positive which usually disappears after the treatment with hyaluronidase.

Electron microscopy has also been used in differentiating mesothelial cells from adenocarcinoma by demonstrating long, thin "bushy" microvilli in the mesotheliomas. Since certain adenocarcinomas can possess short microvilli, some authors suggested that only microvilli with a length/diameter ratio of 15 or above should be considered to be strongly supportive of mesothelioma. However, poorly differentiated epithelial and sarcomatous mesotheliomas may lack microvilli. Furthermore, the availability of adequate material, sizable costs, and long turnaround

**Table 12.3** Markers for mesothelial cells and adenocarcinoma

| Positive mesothelial markers | Positive adenocarcinoma markers |
| --- | --- |
| Calretinin | CEA |
| CK 5/6 | B72.3 |
| N-cadherin | CD15 (leuM1) |
| Mesothelin | BER-EP4 |
|  | MOC-31 |
|  | CA125 |
|  | E-Cadherin |
| WT-1 | WT-1 |

times limit the universal implementation of this technique.

Immunohistochemistry is the most commonly employed ancillary technique. Table 12.3 summarizes markers for mesothelial cells and adenocarcinoma.

### 12.4.4.2 Positive Mesothelial Markers

Calretinin is a 29 kDa protein, member of a large family of calcium-binding proteins. It is the best and most frequently used marker for mesothelioma available. Not only stains epithelial MM, but also some sarcomatoid MM. Calretinin is positive in 80–100% of the epithelial mesotheliomas and 8% of adenocarcinomas of various origins (usually weak and focal). The type of staining found in MM by calretinin varies according to the different studies from finely granular and cytoplasmic staining (nuclei negative) to positive nuclear and cytoplasmic staining. In most recent reports, the staining in MM is strong and diffuse and occurs in both the cytoplasm and the nucleus. Calretinin expression also occurs in squamous cell carcinomas.

Cytokeratin 5/6 is one of the most sensitive of the positive mesotheliomas markers. It is expressed in over 90–100% of epithelial mesotheliomas, but is absent in sarcomatoid mesotheliomas. Cytokeratin 5/6 expression commonly occurs in squamous carcinomas and can be seen in a minority of adenocarcinomas where the staining if focal and limited to few cells (<5% of the tumor cells). In mesothelial cells, the staining of CK 5/6 is strong and diffuse throughout the cytoplasm.

Wilm's tumor gene (WT-1) is a nuclear DNA-binding protein. It is a tumor suppressor gene and is expressed in mesangial cells of the kidney, Sertoli cells of the testis, ovarian stromal cells and surface epithelium, and reactive mesothelial cells as well as in some adenocarcinomas, particularly papillary serous carcinomas. Positive nuclear staining is seen in 75–93% of the MM. It is not useful in separating MM form serous carcinomas of the ovary and peritoneum.

Mesothelin is a 40-kDa surface glycoprotein of unknown function that is strongly expressed in normal mesothelial cells and MM. Mesothelin is a very sensitive positive marker for MM (100%), but the specificity is low (positivity in 50% of ovarian adenocarcinomas) In addition, it has been shown that mesothelin is strongly expressed in serous carcinoma of the ovary, pancreatic adenocarcinoma and some squamous carcinomas.

N-cadherin is one of the most recently recognized positive markers for MM. It is an adhesion protein that is found in nerve cells, developing muscle cells and mesothelial cells. Positive staining is usually noted along the cell membrane. Reported positivity with N-cadherin for MM varies from 77 to 100%, whereas only 19–30% of the adenocarcinomas were positive. N-cadherin is commonly expressed in papillary serous and endometrioid carcinomas of the ovary. This marker has no value in differentiating these two tumors from mesotheliomas.

### 12.4.4.3 Positive Adenocarcinoma Markers

CEA is the first marker to be accepted as being useful in distinguishing MM from adenocarcinoma. Eighty-eight percent of the lung adenocarcinomas express CEA, while mesotheliomas are almost invariably negative. The staining is cytoplasmic with accentuation of the cell membrane. It should be emphasized that this marker is expressed in only 20% of the serous carcinomas. The best results are obtained with monoclonal antibodies. Antigen retrieval results are stronger and more diffuse staining of the adenocarcinomas. CEA is a highly sensitive and specific marker for adenocarcinoma and continues to be one of the best negative mesothelioma markers. Its value is limited for discriminating MM form serous carcinoma of the ovary and peritoneum because less than half of the latter tumors expressed this marker.

MOC-31 is a monoclonal antibody against a glycoprotein generated using the GLS-1 small cell lung carcinoma cell line. It is the best markers currently available for distinguishing M from adenocarcinoma. Strong and diffuse (>50% of the tumor cells) cytoplasmic staining is seen in 95% of ovary adenocarcinomas. Positive staining for MOC-31 has been reported in 5–10% of the MM; however, staining is usually focal and weak. MOC-31, therefore, is a very helpful marker and a strong diffuse positive staining is against the diagnosis of MM.

B72.3 is a monoclonal antibody against a glycoprotein (TAG-72) present in breast cancer cells and is present in 84% of the lung adenocarcinomas and 87% of the serous carcinomas. Positive staining has been reported in 2–5% of the MM. When it occurs in MM, it is usually focal and confined to a few cells. A coarse granular cytoplasmic staining with apical intensification is characteristic for this marker.

LeuM1 (CD15) is one the earliest markers in the diagnosis of mesothelioma. It is reported to bind to a specific sugar moiety also known as X-hapten that is found in the glycolipids. Most adenocarcinomas exhibit a granular cytoplasmic staining with occasional membrane accentuation. Staining in MM is usually focal and weak.

Ber-EP4 is a monoclonal antibody that was raised using breast cancer cell lines MCF-7 as immunogen. It recognizes two glycoproteins present on the cell membrane of most normal and neoplastic epithelial cells. When positive, adenocarcinomas show a strong and diffuse cytoplasmic and cell membrane staining for BerEP4. The percentage of positivity for Ber-EP4 in ovarian adenocarcinomas is 30–50%.

From a practical point of view, a panel of four markers (two positive and two negative) usually allow for the distinction between epithelioid MM and adenocarcinoma. In our experience, we use calretinin and CK 5/6 as the positive markers for MM and the CEA, B72.3, and/or MOC-31 as the adenocarcinoma markers.

### 12.4.4.4 Reactive Mesothelial Cells Versus Malignant Mesothelial Cells

Ancillary studies employed to differentiate reactive mesothelial cells from mesothelioma, particularly well differentiated one include electron microscopy (EM), DNA ploidy measurement, and immunohistochemistry. EM is helpful in differentiating adenocarcinoma from mesothelial cells. However, it cannot separate benign from neoplastic mesothelial cells. In a study comparing the ploidy of benign effusions with that of mesothelioma, all benign effusions were diploid, whereas 53% of mesotheliomas were aneuploid. However, current literature does not support the routine use of ploidy measurement in clinical setting.

Immunohistochemistry is the most commonly employed ancillary studies in clinical setting.

Majority of the antimesothelial antibodies, such as calretinin, cytokeratin 5/6, thrombomodulin, N-cadherin, and HBME-1 stain both benign and neoplastic mesothelial cells. Mesothelioma cells often demonstrate strong membrane staining for EMA but not in reactive mesothelial cells. Desmin positivity is not only noted in 84% cases of benign/reactive effusion, but also in 22% of mesothelioma. Others have reported that over 50% of mesotheliomas and <10% of the reactive mesothelial cells demonstrate nuclear staining with p53. The staining in reactive mesothelial cells is often weak and limited to occasional cells.

## Suggested Reading

Clement PB, Young RH. Atlas of Gynecologic Surgical Pathology. 2nd Edition. Saunders, Philadelphia, PA, 2008.

Kurman R. Blaustein's Pathology of the Female Genital Tract. 5th Edition. Springer, Berlin, 2002.

Lin O. Challenges in the interpretation of peritoneal cytologic specimens. Arch. Pathol. Lab. Med. 2009; 133:739–42.

Obermair A, et al. Peritoneal cytology: impact on disease-free survival in clinical stage I endometrioid adenocarcinoma of the uterus. Cancer Lett. 2001; 164:105–10.

Patel NP, et al. Cytomorphologic features of primary peritoneal mesothelioma in effusion, washing, and fine-needle aspiration biopsy specimens: examination of 49 cases at one institution, including post-intraperitoneal hyperthermic chemotherapy findings. Am. J. Clin. Pathol. 2007; 128:414–22.

Sadeghi S, Ylagan LR. Pelvic washing cytology in serous borderline tumors of the ovary using ThinPrep: are there cytologic clues to detecting tumor cells? Diagn. Cytopathol. 2004; 30:313–9.

# Appendix

## VULVA STAGING FORM

| CLINICAL<br>*Extent of disease before<br>any treatment* | STAGE CATEGORY DEFINITIONS | | PATHOLOGIC<br>*Extent of disease during and from<br>surgery* |
|---|---|---|---|
| ☐ y clinical– staging completed after neoadjuvant therapy but before subsequent surgery | **TUMOR SIZE:** _____ | **LATERALITY:**<br>☐ left  ☐ right  ☐ bilateral | ☐ y pathologic – staging completed after neoadjuvant therapy AND subsequent surgery |

| TNM<br>CATEGORY | FIGO<br>STAGE | PRIMARY TUMOR (T) | TNM<br>CATEGORY | FIGO<br>STAGE |
|---|---|---|---|---|
| ☐ TX | | Primary tumor cannot be assessed | ☐ TX | |
| ☐ T0 | | No evidence of primary tumor | ☐ T0 | |
| ☐ Tis | * | Carcinoma *in situ* (preinvasive carcinoma) | ☐ Tis | * |
| ☐ T1a | IA | Lesions ≤ 2 cm in size, confined to the vulva or perineum and with stromal invasion ≤ 1.0 mm** | ☐ T1a | IA |
| ☐ T1b | IB | Lesions >2 cm in size **or** any size with stromal invasion >1.0 mm, confined to the vulva or perineum | ☐ T1b | IB |
| ☐ T2*** | II | Tumor of any size with extension to adjacent perineal structures (Lower/distal 1/3 urethra, lower/distal 1/3 vagina, anal involvement) | ☐ T2*** | II |
| ☐ T3**** | IVA | Tumor of any size with extension to any of the following: upper/proximal 2/3 of urethra, upper/proximal 2/3 vagina, bladder mucosa, rectal mucosa, or fixed to pelvic bone, | ☐ T3**** | IVA |

* FIGO staging no longer includes Stage 0 (Tis).

** The depth of invasion is defined as the measurement of the tumor from the epithelial-stromal junction of the adjacent most superficial dermal papilla to the deepest point of invasion.

*** FIGO uses the classification T2/T3. This is defined as T2 in TNM.

**** FIGO uses the classification T4. This is defined as T3 in TNM.

| TNM<br>CATEGORY | FIGO<br>STAGE | REGIONAL LYMPH NODES (N) | TNM<br>CATEGORY | FIGO<br>STAGE |
|---|---|---|---|---|
| ☐ NX | | Regional lymph nodes cannot be assessed | ☐ NX | |
| ☐ N0 | | No regional lymph node metastasis | ☐ N0 | |
| ☐ N1 | | One or two regional lymph node with the following features | ☐ N1 | |
| ☐ N1a | IIIA | One or two lymph node metastasis each 5 mm or less | ☐ N1a | IIIA |
| ☐ N1b | IIIA | One lymph node metastases 5 mm or greater | ☐ N1b | IIIB |
| ☐ N2 | IIIB | Regional lymph node metastasis with the following features: | ☐ N2 | IIIB |
| ☐ N2a | IIIB | Three or more lymph node metastases each less than 5 mm | ☐ N2a | IIIB |
| ☐ N2b | IIIB | Two or more lymph node metastases 5 mm or greater | ☐ N2b | IIIB |
| ☐ N2c | IIIC | Lymph node metastasis with extracapsular spread | ☐ N2c | IIIC |
| ☐ N3 | IVA | Fixed or ulcerated regional lymph node metastasis | ☐ N3 | IVA |

An effort should be made to describe the site and laterality of lymph node metastases.

| TNM<br>CATEGORY | FIGO<br>STAGE | DISTANT METASTASIS (M) | TNM<br>CATEGORY | FIGO<br>STAGE |
|---|---|---|---|---|
| ☐ M0 | | No distant metastasis (no pathologic M0; use clinical M to complete stage group) | | |
| ☐ M1 | IVB | Distant metastasis (including pelvic lymph node metastasis) | ☐ M1 | IVB |

| HOSPITAL NAME/ADDRESS | PATIENT NAME/INFORMATION |
|---|---|
| | |

*(continued on next page)*

## VAGINA STAGING FORM

| CLINICAL<br>*Extent of disease before<br>any treatment* | STAGE CATEGORY DEFINITIONS | | PATHOLOGIC<br>*Extent of disease during and from<br>surgery* |
|---|---|---|---|
| ☐ y clinical – staging completed<br>after neoadjuvant therapy but<br>before subsequent surgery | **TUMOR SIZE:** _____ | **LATERALITY:**<br>☐ left ☐ right ☐ bilateral | ☐ y pathologic – staging completed<br>after neoadjuvant therapy AND<br>subsequent surgery |

| TNM<br>CATEGORY | FIGO<br>STAGE | PRIMARY TUMOR (T) | | TNM<br>CATEGORY | FIGO<br>STAGE |
|---|---|---|---|---|---|
| ☐ TX | | Primary tumor cannot be assessed | | ☐ TX | |
| ☐ T0 | | No evidence of primary tumor | | ☐ T0 | |
| ☐ Tis | * | Carcinoma *in situ* | | ☐ Tis | * |
| ☐ T1 | I | Tumor confined to vagina | | ☐ T1 | I |
| ☐ T2 | II | Tumor invades paravaginal tissues but not to pelvic wall | | ☐ T2 | II |
| ☐ T3 | III | Tumor extends to pelvic wall** | | ☐ T3 | III |
| ☐ T4 | IVA | Tumor invades mucosa of the bladder or rectum and/or extends beyond the true<br>pelvis (bullous edema is not sufficient evidence to classify a tumor as T4) | | ☐ T4 | IVA |
| | | *FIGO staging no longer includes Stage 0 (Tis). | | | |
| | | **Pelvic wall is defined as muscle, fascia, neurovascular structures, or skeletal<br>portions of the bony pelvis. | | | |

| TNM<br>CATEGORY | FIGO<br>STAGE | REGIONAL LYMPH NODES (N) | | TNM<br>CATEGORY | FIGO<br>STAGE |
|---|---|---|---|---|---|
| ☐ NX | | Regional lymph nodes cannot be assessed | | ☐ NX | |
| ☐ N0 | | No regional lymph node metastasis | | ☐ N0 | |
| ☐ N1 | III | Pelvic or inguinal lymph node metastasis | | ☐ N1 | III |

| TNM<br>CATEGORY | FIGO<br>STAGE | DISTANT METASTASIS (M) | | TNM<br>CATEGORY | FIGO<br>STAGE |
|---|---|---|---|---|---|
| ☐ M0 | | No distant metastasis  (no pathologic M0; use clinical M to complete stage group) | | ☐ M0 | |
| ☐ M1 | IVB | Distant metastasis | | ☐ M1 | IVB |

## ANATOMIC STAGE • PROGNOSTIC GROUP

| | CLINICAL | | | | | PATHOLOGIC | | |
|---|---|---|---|---|---|---|---|---|
| **GROUP** | **T** | **N** | **M** | | **GROUP** | **T** | **N** | **M** |
| ☐ 0 | Tis | N0 | M0 | | ☐ 0 | Tis | N0 | M0 |
| ☐ I | T1 | N0 | M0 | | ☐ I | T1 | N0 | M0 |
| ☐ II | T2 | N0 | M0 | | ☐ II | T2 | N0 | M0 |
| ☐ III | T1–T3 | N1 | M0 | | ☐ III | T1–T3 | N1 | M0 |
| | T3 | N0 | M0 | | | T3 | N0 | M0 |
| ☐ IVA | T4 | Any N | M0 | | ☐ IVA | T4 | Any N | M0 |
| ☐ IVB | Any T | Any N | M1 | | ☐ IVB | Any T | Any N | M1 |

*FIGO no longer includes Stage 0 (Tis).

☐ Stage unknown

*FIGO no longer includes Stage 0 (Tis).

☐ Stage unknown

| HOSPITAL NAME/ADDRESS | PATIENT NAME/INFORMATION |
|---|---|
| | |

*(continued on next page)*

# CERVIX UTERI STAGING FORM

| CLINICAL Extent of disease before any treatment | STAGE CATEGORY DEFINITIONS | | PATHOLOGIC Extent of disease through completion of definitive surgery |
|---|---|---|---|
| ☐ y clinical – staging completed after neoadjuvant therapy but before subsequent surgery | TUMOR SIZE: _____ | LATERALITY: ☐ left ☐ right ☐ bilateral | ☐ y pathologic – staging completed after neoadjuvant therapy AND subsequent surgery |

| TNM CATEGORY | FIGO STAGE | PRIMARY TUMOR (T) | TNM CATEGORY | FIGO STAGE |
|---|---|---|---|---|
| ☐ TX | | Primary tumor cannot be assessed | ☐ TX | |
| ☐ T0 | | No evidence of primary tumor | ☐ T0 | |
| ☐ Tis | * | Carcinoma *in situ* (preinvasive carcinoma) | ☐ Tis | * |
| ☐ T1 | I | Cervical carcinoma confined to uterus (extension to corpus should be disregarded) | ☐ T1 | I |
| ☐ T1a** | IA | Invasive carcinoma diagnosed only by microscopy. Stromal invasion with a maximum depth of 5.0 mm measured from the base of the epithelium and a horizontal spread of 7.0 mm or less. Vascular space involvement, venous or lymphatic, does not affect classification | ☐ T1a** | IA |
| ☐ T1a1 | IA1 | Measured stromal invasion 3.0 mm or less in depth and 7.0 mm or less in horizontal spread | ☐ T1a1 | IA1 |
| ☐ T1a2 | IA2 | Measured stromal invasion more than 3.0 mm and not more than 5.0 mm with a horizontal spread 7.0 mm or less | ☐ T1a2 | IA2 |
| ☐ T1b | IB | Clinically visible lesion confined to the cervix or microscopic lesion greater than T1a/IA2 | ☐ T1b | IB |
| ☐ T1b1 | IB1 | Clinically visible lesion 4.0 cm or less in greatest dimension | ☐ T1b1 | IB1 |
| ☐ T1b2 | IB2 | Clinically visible lesion more than 4.0 cm in greatest dimension | ☐ T1b2 | IB2 |
| ☐ T2 | II | Cervical carcinoma invades beyond uterus but not to pelvic wall or to lower third of vagina | ☐ T2 | II |
| ☐ T2a | IIA | Tumor without parametrial invasion | ☐ T2a | IIA |
| ☐ T2a1 | IIA1 | Clinically visible lesion 4.0 cm or less in greatest dimension | ☐ T2a1 | IIA1 |
| ☐ T2a2 | IIA2 | Clinically visible lesion more than 4.0 cm in greatest dimension | ☐ T2a2 | IIA2 |
| ☐ T2b | IIB | Tumor with parametrial invasion | ☐ T2b | IIB |
| ☐ T3 | III | Tumor extends to pelvic wall and/or involves lower third of vagina, and/or causes hydronephrosis or non-functioning kidney | ☐ T3 | III |
| ☐ T3a | IIIA | Tumor involves lower third of vagina, no extension to pelvic wall | ☐ T3a | IIIA |
| ☐ T3b | IIIB | Tumor extends to pelvic wall and/or causes hydronephrosis or non-functioning kidney | ☐ T3b | IIIB |
| ☐ T4 | IVA | Tumor invades mucosa of bladder or rectum, and/or extends beyond true pelvis (bullous edema is not sufficient to classify a tumor as T4) | ☐ T4 | IVA |

* FIGO staging no longer includes Stage 0 (Tis)

** All macroscopically visible lesions—even with superficial invasion—are T1b/IB.

| TNM CATEGORY | FIGO STAGE | REGIONAL LYMPH NODES (N) | TNM CATEGORY | FIGO STAGE |
|---|---|---|---|---|
| ☐ NX | | Regional lymph nodes cannot be assessed | ☐ NX | |
| ☐ N0 | | No regional lymph node metastasis | ☐ N0 | |
| ☐ N1 | IIIB | Reginal lymph node metastasis | ☐ N1 | IIIB |

## CORPUS UTERI CARCINOMA STAGING FORM
### (Carcinosarcomas should be staged as carcinomas)

| CLINICAL<br>*Extent of disease before any treatment* | STAGE CATEGORY DEFINITIONS | | PATHOLOGIC<br>*Extent of disease through completion of definitive surgery* |
|---|---|---|---|
| ☐ y clinical – staging completed after neoadjuvant therapy but before subsequent surgery | TUMOR SIZE: _____ | LATERALITY:<br>☐ left  ☐ right  ☐ bilateral | ☐ y pathologic – staging completed after neoadjuvant therapy AND subsequent surgery |

| TNM CATEGORY | FIGO STAGE | PRIMARY TUMOR (T) | | TNM CATEGORY | FIGO STAGE |
|---|---|---|---|---|---|
| ☐ TX | | Primary tumor cannot be assessed | | ☐ TX | |
| ☐ T0 | | No evidence of primary tumor | | ☐ T0 | |
| ☐ Tis | * | Carcinoma *in situ* (preinvasive carcinoma) | | ☐ Tis | * |
| ☐ T1 | I | Tumor confined to corpus uteri | | ☐ T1 | I |
| ☐ T1a | IA | Tumor limited to endometrium or invades less than one-half of the myometrium | | ☐ T1a | IA |
| ☐ T1b | IB | Tumor invades one-half or more of the myometrium | | ☐ T1b | IB |
| ☐ T2 | II | Tumor invades stromal connective tissue of the cervix but does not extend beyond uterus** | | ☐ T2 | II |
| ☐ T3a | IIIA | Tumor involves serosa and/or adnexa (direct extension or metastasis) | | ☐ T3a | IIIA |
| ☐ T3b | IIIB | Vaginal involvement (direct extension or metastasis) or parametrial involvement | | ☐ T3b | IIIB |
| ☐ T4 | IVA | Tumor invades bladder mucosa and/or bowel mucosa (bullous edema is not sufficient to classify a tumor as T4) | | ☐ T4 | IVA |
| | | * FIGO staging no longer includes Stage 0 (Tis) | | | |
| | | ** Endocervical glandular involvement only should be considered as stage I and not Stage II. | | | |

| TNM CATEGORY | FIGO STAGE | REGIONAL LYMPH NODES (N) | | TNM CATEGORY | FIGO STAGE |
|---|---|---|---|---|---|
| ☐ NX | | Regional lymph nodes cannot be assessed | | ☐ NX | |
| ☐ N0 | | No regional lymph node metastasis | | ☐ N0 | |
| ☐ N1 | IIIC1 | Regional lymph node metastasis to pelvic lymph nodes | | ☐ N1 | IIIC1 |
| ☐ N2 | IIIC2 | Regional lymph node metastasis to para-aortic lymph nodes, with or without positive pelvic lymph nodes | | ☐ N2 | IIIC2 |

| TNM CATEGORY | FIGO STAGE | DISTANT METASTASIS (M) | | TNM CATEGORY | FIGO STAGE |
|---|---|---|---|---|---|
| ☐ M0 | | No distant metastasis (no pathologic M0; use clinical M to complete stage group) | | | |
| ☐ M1 | IVB | Distant metastasis (includes metastasis to inguinal lymph nodes intraperitoneal disease, or lung, liver, or bone. It excludes metastasis to para-aortic lymph nodes, vagina, pelvic serosa, or adnexa) | | ☐ M1 | IVB |

## GESTATIONAL TROPHOBLASTIC TUMORS STAGING FORM

| CLINICAL<br>Extent of disease before<br>any treatment | STAGE CATEGORY DEFINITIONS | | PATHOLOGIC<br>Extent of disease through<br>completion of definitive surgery |
|---|---|---|---|
| ☐ y clinical – staging completed<br>after neoadjuvant therapy but<br>before subsequent surgery | TUMOR SIZE: _____ | LATERALITY:<br>☐ left ☐ right ☐ bilateral | ☐ y pathologic – staging completed<br>after neoadjuvant therapy AND<br>subsequent surgery |

| TNM CATEGORY | FIGO STAGE | PRIMARY TUMOR (T) | | TNM CATEGORY | FIGO STAGE |
|---|---|---|---|---|---|
| ☐ TX | | Primary tumor cannot be assessed | | ☐ TX | |
| ☐ T0 | | No evidence of primary tumor | | ☐ T0 | |
| ☐ T1 | I | Tumor confined to uterus | | ☐ T1 | I |
| ☐ T2 | II | Tumor extends to other genital structures (ovary, tube, vagina, broad ligaments)<br>by metastasis or direct extension | | ☐ T2 | II |

| | | REGIONAL LYMPH NODES (N) | | | |
|---|---|---|---|---|---|
| | | There is no regional nodal designation in the staging of these tumors. Nodal<br>metastases should be classified as metastatic (M1) disease. | | | |

| TNM CATEGORY | FIGO STAGE | DISTANT METASTASIS (M) | | TNM CATEGORY | FIGO STAGE |
|---|---|---|---|---|---|
| ☐ M0 | | No distant metastasis (no pathologic M0; use clinical M to complete stage group) | | ☐ M0 | |
| ☐ M1 | | Distant metastasis | | ☐ M1 | |
| ☐ M1a | III | Lung metastasis | | ☐ M1a | III |
| ☐ M1b | IV | All other distant metastasis | | ☐ M1b | IV |

### ANATOMIC STAGE • PROGNOSTIC GROUPS

| | | CLINICAL | | | | | | PATHOLOGIC | | | |
|---|---|---|---|---|---|---|---|---|---|---|---|
| GROUP | T | N | M | RISK SCORE | | GROUP | T | N | M | RISK SCORE | |
| ☐ I | T1 | | M0 | Unknown | | ☐ I | T1 | | M0 | Unknown | |
| ☐ IA | T1 | | M0 | Low risk | | ☐ IA | T1 | | M0 | Low risk | |
| ☐ IB | T1 | | M0 | High risk | | ☐ IB | T1 | | M0 | High risk | |
| ☐ II | T2 | | M0 | Unknown | | ☐ II | T2 | | M0 | Unknown | |
| ☐ IIA | T2 | | M0 | Low risk | | ☐ IIA | T2 | | M0 | Low risk | |
| ☐ IIB | T2 | | M0 | High risk | | ☐ IIB | T2 | | M0 | High risk | |
| ☐ III | Any T | | M1a | Unknown | | ☐ III | Any T | | M1a | Unknown | |
| ☐ IIIA | Any T | | M1a | Low risk | | ☐ IIIA | Any T | | M1a | Low risk | |
| ☐ IIIB | Any T | | M1a | High risk | | ☐ IIIB | Any T | | M1a | High risk | |
| ☐ IV | Any T | | M1b | Unknown | | ☐ IV | Any T | | M1b | Unknown | |
| ☐ IVA | Any T | | M1b | Low risk | | ☐ IVA | Any T | | M1b | Low risk | |
| ☐ IVB | Any T | | M1b | High risk | | ☐ IVB | Any T | | M1b | High risk | |
| ☐ Stage unknown | | | | | | ☐ Stage unknown | | | | | |

## FALLOPIAN TUBE STAGING FORM

| CLINICAL Extent of disease before any treatment | STAGE CATEGORY DEFINITIONS | | PATHOLOGIC Extent of disease through completion of definitive surgery |
|---|---|---|---|
| ☐ y clinical – staging completed after neoadjuvant therapy but before subsequent surgery | TUMOR SIZE:_____ | LATERALITY: ☐ left ☐ right ☐ bilateral | ☐ y pathologic – staging completed after neoadjuvant therapy AND subsequent surgery |

| TNM CATEGORY | FIGO STAGE | PRIMARY TUMOR (T) | TNM CATEGORY | FIGO STAGE |
|---|---|---|---|---|
| ☐ TX | | Primary tumor cannot be assessed | ☐ TX | |
| ☐ T0 | | No evidence of primary tumor | ☐ T0 | |
| ☐ Tis | * | Carcinoma *in situ* (limited to tubal mucosa) | ☐ Tis | * |
| ☐ T1 | I | Tumor limited to the fallopian tube(s) | ☐ T1 | IA |
| ☐ T1a | IA | Tumor limited to one tube, without penetrating the serosal surface; no ascites | | |
| ☐ T1b | IB | Tumor limited to both tubes, without penetrating the serosal surface; no ascites | ☐ T2 | IB |
| ☐ T1c | IC | Tumor limited to one or both tubes with extension onto or through the tubal serosa, or with malignant cells in ascites or peritoneal washings | ☐ T3 | II |
| ☐ T2 | II | Tumor involves one or both fallopian tubes with pelvic extension | | |
| ☐ T2a | IIA | Extension and/or metastasis to the uterus and/or ovaries | ☐ T4 | IVA |
| ☐ T2b | IIB | Extension to other pelvic structures | | |
| ☐ T2c | IIC | Pelvic extension with malignant cells in ascites or peritoneal washings | | |
| ☐ T3 | III | Tumor involves one or both fallopian tubes, with peritoneal implants outside the pelvis | | |
| ☐ T3a | IIIA | Microscopic peritoneal metastasis outside the pelvis | | |
| ☐ T3b | IIIB | Macroscopic peritoneal metastasis outside the pelvis 2 cm or less in greatest dimension | | |
| ☐ T3c | IIIC | Peritoneal metastasis outside the pelvis and more than 2 cm in diameter | | |
| | | * FIGO no longer includes Stage 0 (Tis) | | |
| | | *Note:* Liver capsule metastasis is T3/Stage III; liver parenchymal metastasis M1/Stage IV. Pleural effusion must have positive cytology for M1/Stage IV. | | |

| TNM CATEGORY | FIGO STAGE | REGIONAL LYMPH NODES (N) | TNM CATEGORY | FIGO STAGE |
|---|---|---|---|---|
| ☐ NX | | Regional lymph nodes cannot be assessed | ☐ NX | |
| ☐ N0 | | No regional lymph node metastasis | ☐ N0 | |
| ☐ N1 | IIIC | Regional lymph node metastasis | ☐ N1 | IIIC |

| TNM CATEGORY | FIGO STAGE | DISTANT METASTASIS (M) | TNM CATEGORY | FIGO STAGE |
|---|---|---|---|---|
| ☐ M0 | | No distant metastasis (no pathologic M0; use clinical M to complete stage group) | | |
| ☐ M1 | IV | Distant metastasis (excludes metastasis within the peritoneal cavity) | ☐ M1 | IV |

## OVARY STAGING FORM

| CLINICAL<br>*Extent of disease before<br>any treatment* | STAGE CATEGORY DEFINITIONS | | PATHOLOGIC<br>*Extent of disease through<br>completion of definitive surgery* |
|---|---|---|---|
| ☐ y clinical – staging completed<br>after neoadjuvant therapy but<br>before subsequent surgery | TUMOR SIZE: _____ | LATERALITY:<br>☐ left  ☐ right  ☐ bilateral | ☐ y pathologic – staging completed<br>after neoadjuvant therapy AND<br>subsequent surgery |

| TNM<br>CATEGORY | FIGO<br>STAGE | PRIMARY TUMOR (T) | TNM<br>CATEGORY | FIGO<br>STAGE |
|---|---|---|---|---|
| ☐ TX | | Primary tumor cannot be assessed | ☐ TX | |
| ☐ T0 | | No evidence of primary tumor | ☐ T0 | |
| ☐ T1 | I | Tumor limited to ovaries (one or both) | ☐ T1 | I |
| ☐ T1a | IA | Tumor limited to one ovary; capsule intact, no tumor on ovarian surface. No malignant cells in ascites or peritoneal washings | ☐ T1a | IA |
| ☐ T1b | IB | Tumor limited to both ovaries; capsules intact, no tumor on ovarian surface. No malignant cells in ascites or peritoneal washings | ☐ T1b | IB |
| ☐ T1c | IC | Tumor limited to one or both ovaries with any of the following: capsule ruptured, tumor on ovarian surface, malignant cells in ascites or peritoneal washings | ☐ T1c | IC |
| ☐ T2 | II | Tumor involves one or both ovaries with pelvic extension and/or implants | ☐ T2 | II |
| ☐ T2a | IIA | Extension and/or implants on uterus and/or tube(s). No malignant cells in ascites or peritoneal washings | ☐ T2a | IIA |
| ☐ T2b | IIB | Extension to and/or implants on other pelvic tissues. No malignant cells in ascites or peritoneal washings | ☐ T2b | IIB |
| ☐ T2c | IIC | Pelvic extension and/or implants (T2a or T2b) with malignant cells in ascites or peritoneal washings | ☐ T2c | IIC |
| ☐ T3 | III | Tumor involves one or both ovaries with microscopically confirmed peritoneal metastasis outside the pelvis | ☐ T3 | III |
| ☐ T3a | IIIA | Microscopic peritoneal metastasis beyond pelvis (no macroscopic tumor) | ☐ T3a | IIIA |
| ☐ T3b | IIIB | Macroscopic peritoneal metastasis beyond pelvis 2 cm or less in greatest dimension | ☐ T3b | IIIB |
| ☐ T3c | IIIC | Peritoneal metastasis beyond pelvis more than 2 cm in greatest dimension and/or regional lymph node metastasis | ☐ T3c | IIIC |
| | | *Note:* Liver capsule metastasis T3/Stage III; liver parenchymal metastasis M1/Stage IV. Pleural effusion must have positive cytology for M1/Stage IV. | | |

| TNM<br>CATEGORY | FIGO<br>STAGE | REGIONAL LYMPH NODES (N) | TNM<br>CATEGORY | FIGO<br>STAGE |
|---|---|---|---|---|
| ☐ NX | | Regional lymph nodes cannot be assessed | ☐ NX | |
| ☐ N0 | | No regional lymph node metastasis | ☐ N0 | |
| ☐ N1 | IIIC | Regional lymph node metastasis | ☐ N1 | IIIC |

| TNM<br>CATEGORY | FIGO<br>STAGE | DISTANT METASTASIS (M) | TNM<br>CATEGORY | FIGO<br>STAGE |
|---|---|---|---|---|
| ☐ M0 | | No distant metastasis  (no pathologic M0; use clinical M to complete stage group) | ☐ M0 | |
| ☐ M1 | IV | Distant metastasis (excludes peritoneal metastasis) | ☐ M1 | IV |

# Index

Printed in the United States of America